EPIDEMIOLOGY FOUNDATIONS

The Science of Public Health

PETER J. FOS

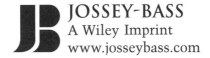
JOSSEY-BASS
A Wiley Imprint
www.josseybass.com

Published by Jossey-Bass

A Wiley Imprint

989 Market Street, San Francisco, CA 94103-1741—www.josseybass.com

Readers should be aware that Internet Web sites offered as citations and/or sources for further information may have changed or disappeared between the time this was written and when it is read.

Limit of Liability/Disclaimer of Warranty: While the publisher and author have used their best efforts in preparing this book, they make no representations or warranties with respect to the accuracy or completeness of the contents of this book and specifically disclaim any implied warranties of merchantability or fitness for a particular purpose. No warranty may be created or extended by sales representatives or written sales materials. The advice and strategies contained herein may not be suitable for your situation. You should consult with a professional where appropriate. Neither the publisher nor author shall be liable for any loss of profit or any other commercial damages, including but not limited to special, incidental, consequential, or other damages.

Jossey-Bass books and products are available through most bookstores. To contact Jossey-Bass directly call our Customer Care Department within the U.S. at 800-956-7739, outside the U.S. at 317-572-3986, or fax 317-572-4002.

Jossey-Bass also publishes its books in a variety of electronic formats. Some content that appears in print may not be available in electronic books.

Library of Congress Cataloging-in-Publication Data

Fos, Peter J.
   Epidemiology foundations : the science of public health / Peter J. Fos.—1st ed.
      p. ; cm.
   Includes bibliographical references and index.
      ISBN 978-0-470-40289-4 (pbk.); ISBN 978-0-470-91070-2 (ebk.); ISBN 978-0-470-91071-9 (ebk.); ISBN 978-0-4709-1072-6 (ebk.)
   1. Epidemiology. I. Title.
   [DNLM: 1. Epidemiologic Methods. 2. Epidemiology. WA 950]
   RA651.F647 2011
   614.4—dc22

                                                                                                    2010040026

Printed in the United States of America

FIRST EDITION

PB Printing   10 9 8 7 6 5 4 3 2 1

For Dylan and Madison Rose
May your futures be bright

CONTENTS

Epidemiology? Many people have heard the term, but few really understand what it is, what it does, and how it influences our daily lives. This book is intended to inform students and practitioners about the vital role of epidemiology in enhancing the health of individuals and communities, to understand how to read and interpret epidemiological studies to become more enlightened citizens, and to understand the global effects of epidemiological studies.

The motivation for this book has developed over the years from the influence of several factors. I have taught epidemiology to graduate students for more than twenty years and have written other textbooks aimed at illustrating the relevance and benefit of epidemiology for specialized uses in health care administration and population health management. Through my years of teaching and writing, I have seen the positive response from students and practitioners to the myriad applications of epidemiology to their respective fields and everyday life. With this in mind, it makes sense to expose young scholars to epidemiology earlier in their intellectual journey. The more people who understand and appreciate the uses of epidemiology, the better chance its application will improve the public's health and well-being.

Another motivation for writing this book is the attention that epidemiology and public health education is receiving from national organizations. National public agencies have been warning that there is a crisis in the shortage of trained and qualified public health workers, especially epidemiologists.[1] There is a movement, which is gaining momentum, to expand the public health education downward from graduate programs to undergraduates, especially into community colleges.[2] This call to action must be met with innovative curricula and instructional resource materials.

Organization

Chapters One and Two lay the foundation to the course by discussing both the historical perspective and future trends of epidemiology. Chapter One, "Why Epidemiology?" introduces the reasons why epidemiology is an important foundation to public health. The chapter presents the role that epidemiology plays in public health. Current and future characteristics of the United States population and of global health threats are presented with an epidemiological perspective. Chapter Two, "History of Epidemiology," continues to provide background information by presenting a historical perspective of the development of epidemiology as the basic science of public health. Past contributors and their influence on the science of epidemiology are discussed.

Chapters Three, Four, and Five discuss health and disease and how they are measured. Chapter Three, "Health and Disease," begins the core discussion of epidemiological principles, along with the foundations of health and disease. The notion of disease causation is discussed and stressed throughout the text. Chapter Four, "Describing Health and Disease," discusses descriptive epidemiology and its uses as an information source and as a precursor to further study and investigation. Emphasis is placed on descriptive variables that are used to explain differences in health and disease in populations. Chapter Five, "Measuring Health and Disease," introduces morbidity and mortality measures. How these measures assist in interpreting disease information is discussed.

Chapters Six and Seven discuss epidemiological studies and how they are used. Chapter Six, "Epidemiological Study Designs: Observational and Experimental Studies," presents study designs used to test hypotheses that result from descriptive information. Observation and experimental designs are introduced. Chapter Seven, "Uses of Epidemiological Studies," covers the evaluation of cause-and-effect relationships between causal factors and diseases. Hypothesis testing and quantification of risk with epidemiological study designs are discussed.

Chapters Eight through Twelve discuss epidemiology from a social and community perspective and global diseases and epidemics. Chapter Eight, "Epidemics," begins the section of the text that focuses on the use of epidemiological principles in everyday life. This chapter discusses epidemics and how they begin and spread. Modes of transmission of infectious agents are described as well as how public health agencies respond to epidemics. Disease surveillance methods, including reportable disease reporting, are presented. Chapter Nine, "Epidemiology and Society," introduces one of the newer epidemiological disciplines. The influence of society and the neighborhoods in which people live on their health is the crux of social epidemiology. Chapter Ten, "Screening for Disease," brings epidemiology to a personal level. Accuracy and precision of screening tests and the evaluation of their results are discussed. Chapter Eleven, "Community Public Health," covers the link connecting epidemiology to improvements in daily life. Public health program planning, implementation, and evaluation are presented. The role of epidemiology in community public health is described through examples of public health programs. Chapter Twelve, "Epidemiology Today," discusses current health and disease concerns, and the pending future impact of current health problems is portrayed from the epidemiological perspective.

Features

Each chapter is supplemented with exercises to aid in understanding the epidemiological principles. These chapter exercises consist of research assignments and problem solving. Most of these exercises are open-ended to challenge the reader to be creative and innovative. In addition, each chapter has a set of multiple-choice, true-or-false, and short-answer review questions. These chapter review questions are intended to provide immediate feedback.

Audience

I anticipate that the primary users of this textbook will be students in high school, community and junior colleges, and four-year colleges and universities. This book can serve as a first resource for students new to epidemiology. One objective is to engage young people in hopes that they will embrace epidemiology as a discipline in which they will continue their study and future work. My hope is that after reading and using this book, students will understand and appreciate the relevance and impact that epidemiology, as the basic science of public health, has on improving health and wellness.

Acknowledgments

This book is a product of more than thirty years of work and study of health and disease. My personal journey has been uncharted at times but thankfully has carried me in a positive and growing direction. I have had many mentors and supporters along the way. Their support has made this journey up to this point one characterized by more ups than downs. Included among my supporters are my students; they have been my true motivation and inspiration. I thank each and every one of you. Finally, I must thank and acknowledge my family. They have allowed me to pursue my career and intellectual pursuits with no complaints, despite the hardships they may have confronted. They have always been my greatest supporters. I must thank my colleagues who have helped me often during my journey, as well as with this book. David J. Fine first convinced me to write books for students. He has been there for me often and is a source of inspiration and encouragement. Peggy Honoré was my student many years ago and now is my friend and colleague. Her encouragement has been invaluable. Miguel Zuniga, also a former student, is now my friend and collaborator in many of my accomplishments. He is a source of technical knowledge and has kept me on task throughout the writing of this book.

Sandra Kiselica edited this book, and her help and recommendations have been invaluable. Her expertise can be seen throughout in the sections that read easiest.

Peter J. Fos

Peter J. Fos is provost and professor of health sciences at the University of Texas at Tyler. He is an internationally known decision scientist and epidemiologist. He earned his doctorate in health care decision analysis from Tulane University Graduate School and his master of public health degree from Tulane University Health Sciences Center, following a career in clinical dentistry. He has spent more than twenty-five years at academic institutions, where he is active in curriculum development in application of epidemiology to management, the practice of managerial epidemiology, clinical effectiveness, public-health practice, health-outcomes research, and terrorism-preparedness planning. He served, briefly, as chief science officer of the Mississippi State Department of Health. He maintains adjunct faculty positions at the University of Southern Mississippi College of Health and the University of Alabama in Birmingham School of Health-Related Professions, and is a visiting scholar at the Medical University of South Carolina, College of Health Professions.

WHY EPIDEMIOLOGY?

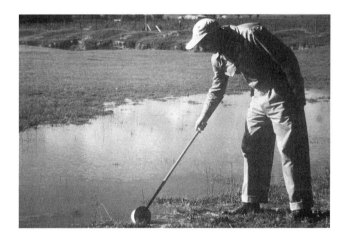

LEARNING OBJECTIVES

On completing this chapter, you will be able to

Define epidemiology
Discuss the concept of populations and population health
Describe population trends and characteristics
Describe global health threats
Discuss the relationship and distinction between public health and medicine

Introduction

Epidemiology is, for most, a word that seems to be from another language. It is certainly not a word we use in everyday conversation. But epidemiology is a science that affects all of us every day of our lives. We shop for food each day with little regard to or worry about whether what we purchase and eat is unsafe. For many of us, smallpox, polio, plague, diphtheria, yellow fever, and cholera are diseases that either we have never heard of or we do not give much thought or attention to. Human immunodeficiency virus (HIV) infection and acquired immunodeficiency syndrome (AIDS) are diseases that are well known, but they are becoming less of a daily concern. New, so-called emerging diseases such as bird flu are now garnering a great deal of our attention.

Public Health and Community Medicine

Before continuing the discussion on "why epidemiology," the concept of public health must be explained further. *Public health* is the science and practice of protecting and improving the health of a community. This can be done with preventive medicine, health education, the control of communicable diseases, the use of sanitary measures, and the monitoring of environmental conditions. Public health is concerned with the health of the community as a whole. In other words, public health and community health are synonymous.

Public health is focused on three areas: assessment and monitoring of health and disease, development of public health policies that assist in addressing health problems, and allowing for access to public health care services. These public health care services include disease prevention, health education, and health promotion. Often public health services are considered to be the same as medical care services because of the assumed similarities. The distinction is that public health services are focused on populations, not individuals. It is true that populations are made up of individuals, so public health acknowledges the importance of the welfare of individuals, but the focus of services is on larger populations. Public health services are centered on diagnosing and monitoring health issues and providing health education and health promotion services to communities.

An example of this communitywide perspective of public health is considered an accomplishment. Public health is concerned with immunization for preventable disease, such as smallpox, poliomyelitis, measles, rubella, tetanus, diphtheria, and *Haemophilus influenzae* type b. Since immunization programs (also referred to as vaccination programs) were established, smallpox has been eradicated, poliomyelitis has been eliminated in the United States, and the other diseases are now under control. Other infectious diseases (cholera, tuberculosis, and sexually transmitted diseases) also are under control, in part due to the efforts of public health agencies and programs.

Is public health the same as medicine? Despite the fact that medical and public health services both seek to improve health, they are not the same. Two easy-to-remember differences are (1) public health services are directed at populations, and medical services are focused on the individual; and (2) public health services are mostly concerned with the prevention of disease whereas medical services are concerned with the diagnosis and treatment of disease. Public health and medicine are different, but they have the same objective of improving health and eliminating disease.

Definition of Epidemiology

Epidemiology is a word with Greek origins: from the Greek prefix *epi*, meaning "on, upon, or befall"; the Greek root *demos*, meaning "the people"; and the Greek suffix *logos*," meaning "the study of." In other words, epidemiology studies that which befalls on people, which is disease. The word epidemiology was first used in the 1700s to describe the science and methods used to study epidemics. In the twentieth century, with the decline of infectious diseases, epidemiology expanded to study more than epidemics. This decline in infectious diseases can be attributed to improvements in nutrition, sanitation, and general living conditions that in part resulted from public health interventions. Of course, these public health interventions were established using information provided by epidemiology.

Given this new need for *epidemiology*, it has been defined as the study of the distribution and determinants of health-related states or events in specified populations and the application of this study to control health problems.[1] This means that epidemiology is used to identify the diseases in a population and to understand why these diseases exist. Another often-used definition is that epidemiology is the study of the distribution and determinants of health-related states and events in *defined* populations and the application of this study to the control of health problems.[2]

The Greek root of epidemiology and the two definitions have a common theme, namely, the people. The people are considered as a group, which is referred to as a *population*. This population-centered nature of epidemiology leads to one of the differences between public health services and medical services. Populations are groups of people who share some common characteristics. These characteristics are personal (age, sex, race, health behaviors), geographical (live in the same neighborhood, city, region, country, continent), and time. Populations may be large groups of people (population of the United States) or small groups (people in a neighborhood or in a factory).

Epidemiology is the study of factors affecting the health and illness of populations. It serves as the foundation of interventions made in the interest of public health and preventive medicine. It is considered a cornerstone method of public health research and is highly regarded in medicine for identifying risk factors for disease and determining the best treatment approaches to clinical practice. Epidemiology is considered by many to be a critical branch of public health. In fact, it is often referred to as the basic science of public health.

Epidemiology provides a framework of methods and principles from which information can be reviewed and analyzed in a way that public health problems can be identified and addressed. The epidemiological methods allow for disease definition as well as classification, identification, and planning for disease control measures. Epidemiology also provides the way to understand the relationship between the presence of factors that cause disease, called *causal factors*, and the development of disease (for example, smoking and heart disease).

Epidemiologists are the people who work every day using epidemiological principles and methods to make our lives better. Epidemiologists identify, measure, count, and control diseases, injuries, and causes of death. They also look for connections between disease and genetic, environmental, and behavioral factors. Once these connections are established, epidemiologists plan and develop interventions to prevent disease and promote health. This process of identifying connections and developing interventions is how epidemiology touches our lives in a positive way every day.

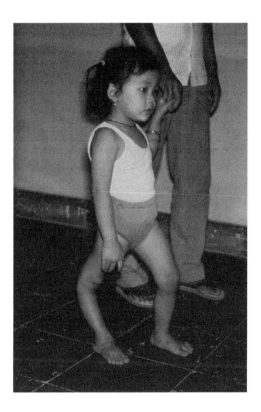

Let's discuss some specific examples of how epidemiology has affected public health. In general terms, most of the significant improvements in the health of the people in the United States can be traced to accomplishments of public health.

An example of how public health policy improved the health and well-being of large groups of people happened in the United States in 1955. At that time, results of field tests of the polio vaccine were announced indicating that an inactivated poliovirus could produce immunity. Within days of this announcement, a national vaccination program was implemented. Today, polio has been eradicated from the United States.

Another accomplishment of public health initiatives with long-term beneficial effects is the identification of the relationship between cigarette smoking and

FIGURE 1.1: Cigarette smoking in the United States, 1965 to 2005

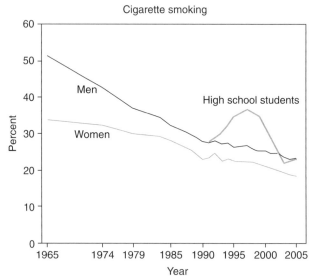

Source: CDC/NCHS, *Health, United States, 2009*, Figure 6. Data from the National Health Interview Survey and the Youth Risk Behavior Survey.

lung cancer and heart disease. Public health and epidemiological reports were instrumental in alerting people to the hazards of cigarette smoking, which led to the warning on cigarette packages from the U.S. Surgeon General. Public health, using epidemiological information as support, has worked hard in the past few decades to decrease the number of smokers in the United States. Figure 1.1 shows the results of this effort.

Figure 1.1 shows that the percentage of people who smoke has drastically decreased since 1965. This reduction has been most significant in men. In 1965 more than 50 percent of men in the United States were smokers. By 2005 the percentage dropped to less than 30 percent. Perhaps the best news is the decrease in the percentage of pregnant smokers. Smoking during pregnancy has been associated with infants with low birth weight and other associated health problems. Smoking among high school students is still a concern, but tobacco cessation efforts have targeted this group for the past few years.

It is interesting to note the decline in heart disease, which in part is due to smoking cessation programs. Figure 1.2 shows the leading causes of death from 1965 to 2006. Overall cancer rates have not changed since 1965, but lung cancer

FIGURE 1.2: Leading causes of death, United States, 1950 to 2004

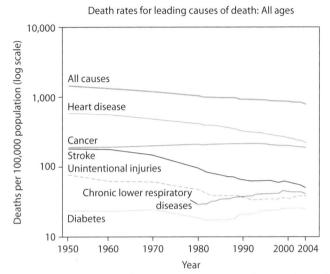

Source: CDC/NCHS, *Health, United States, 2009*, Figure 18. Data from the National Vital Statistics System.

deaths have declined. Deaths due to stroke have decreased dramatically, which can be attributed to tobacco cessation programs. Also, because of public health awareness and legislation, unintentional motor vehicle injuries have decreased due to mandatory seat beat usage and protective restraints.

Other accomplishments of public health include global eradication of smallpox and establishing the relationship between Reye's syndrome and aspirin. The eradication of smallpox may be one of the greatest accomplishments of medicine and public health. Smallpox is a serious, contagious, and often fatal infectious disease. In the past, it killed almost 30 percent of infected people, and it left scars on the skin of those who survived. No vaccine or treatment existed until the end of the eighteenth century, when Edward Jenner introduced the smallpox vaccination. The last case of smallpox in the United States was in 1949, and the last naturally occurring case in the world was in Somalia in 1977.[3]

Reye's syndrome is a disease that affects all organs of the body but is particularly damaging to the liver and brain. The exact cause of Reye's syndrome is unknown, but it has been shown to be associated with aspirin usage. Cases are most often seen in January–March each year. An epidemic of flu or chickenpox is commonly followed by an increase in the number of cases of Reye's syndrome.[4]

Epidemiology had a major role in the investigation of smallpox and Reye's syndrome. In fact, epidemiology is responsible for discovering the cause, and for developing control measures for other diseases such as Legionnaire's disease. Legionnaire's disease acquired its name in July 1976 when an outbreak of pneumonia occurred among people attending a convention of the American Legion in Philadelphia. On January 18, 1977, the causative agent was identified as a previously unknown bacterium, subsequently named *Legionella pneumophila.* An estimated 8,000 to 18,000 people get legionellosis in the United States each year. Some people can be infected with the *Legionella* bacterium and have only mild symptoms or no illness at all. When outbreaks do occur, they are usually in the summer and early autumn, though cases may occur at any time of the year.[5]

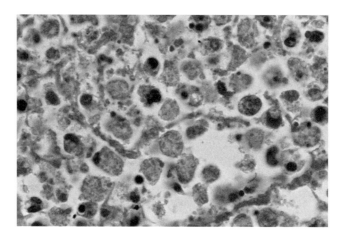

Another well-known accomplishment of epidemiology and public health is the work with AIDS. AIDS is the final stage of HIV infection. HIV attacks the body's immune system. Our bodies' immune system fights infections. HIV finds and destroys a white blood cell (called a T-cell) that is important for the immune system to fight infections. For someone who has HIV infection, it can takes years before they have AIDS. AIDS is a disease in which a person has enough of a weakened immune system that the body has trouble fighting off infection. It was through the use of epidemiological methods that the HIV infection and AIDS were identified, along with the factors that were associated with a person's susceptibility. These factors were found to include both behavioral and social causes.

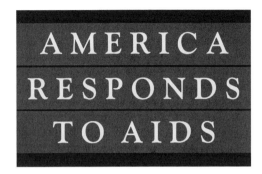

Public health continues to make major improvements in health by controlling epidemics, providing safe water and food, and establishing maternal and child health services. As will be discussed throughout this book, public health, with the help of the science of epidemiology, has done such a remarkable job of preventing countless deaths and improving the quality of life that many of us take it for granted. One reason to study public health and epidemiology is to become aware of how our daily lives are affected by public health and epidemiology. According to the Institute of Medicine in the report, *The Future of Public Health*, "An impossible responsibility has been placed on America's public health agencies: to serve as stewards of the basic health needs of entire populations, but at the same time avert impending disasters and provide personal health care to those rejected by the rest of the health system. The wonder is not that American public health has problems, but that so much has been done so well, and with so little."[6]

Population Health

The health of a population is a prime focus of epidemiology and public health. The health of populations was first studied in the seventeenth century. A population is not a fixed, standard number of people but is a specific group under study because of some common traits. These traits are associated with disease exposures, including the effect of social conditions. Often when looking at a population, the total population is the target, but smaller parts of that population may be studied (these are called *subpopulations*). For example, the students in a school constitute a population whereas the students in a classroom are a subpopulation.

Usually populations are defined by geographical boundaries—for example, residents in a country, regions of a country, states, cities, and sections of a city. This is done because people in specific geographical locations have common traits, including age, sex, race, and other characteristics. Geographical populations are studied because it is easy to gather the necessary data about the populations. This is due, in part, to the fact that geographically defined areas are related to political and governmental units as well as public health agencies.

A goal of epidemiology is to identify and prevent factors that cause disease in populations. To do this, epidemiology starts its study at the population level and then addresses the identified determinants of health and disease at this level.[7] Epidemiology studies populations that are made up of individuals, but the focus remains on the population.[8] So it is important to understand the relationship between disease and its causal factors at both the population and individual person levels.[9]

It is also important to remember that populations differ. Populations can be divided into several subpopulations based on many factors, including demographics. These different subpopulations will have different health care needs and will use health care services in different ways.[10]

It is now known that social conditions, conditions that people live in, can affect a population's health. Different socioenvironmental exposures are related to differing physical and mental health outcomes. Epidemiology studies the affect of social conditions in its branch science called *social epidemiology*. Social epidemiology studies how society and social organization influence the health and wellness of people in populations. Social epidemiology tries to explain the connection between exposure to social characteristics of the environment and its effects on health, with the hopeful result of a better understanding of how, where, and why social inequalities affect health.

Population Trends

Epidemiology is a science that studies populations. The makeup of a population directly affects health and disease. If you can understand characteristics of a population, and if the population is changing, then it becomes easier to plan for disease prevention and treatment.

The population of the United States has been increasing for the past few decades. This increase is expected to continue to at least the year 2050. Figure

FIGURE 1.3: Projected population growth, 2010 to 2050, in the United States

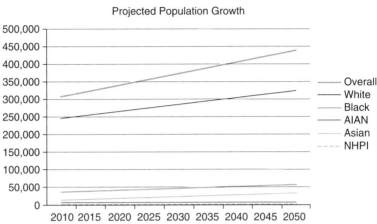

Projected Population Growth

Source: U.S. Census Bureau, Population Division, Projection of the Population and Components of Change for the United States: 2010–2050.
AIAN refers to American Indians and Alaska Natives
NHPI refers to Native Hawaiians and Pacific Islanders

1.3 shows the projected population growth from 2010 to 2050. Overall the population is expected to increase from just over 300 million people to almost 450 million. Growth is expected among all races—whites, blacks, American Indians and Alaska Natives, Asians, Native Hawaiians and Pacific Islanders.

As the population grows over the next forty years, the age percentages will change slightly, with an obvious aging of the population. The percentage of people younger than forty-four years will decrease, and the percentage will increase for people aged forty-five years and older. The percentage of people younger than eighteen years will decrease from 28 percent to 23 percent. Among people aged eighteen to forty-four, the percentage will decrease from 40 percent to 34 percent. The percentage of people older than seventy-five years will more than double from 4 percent to 11 percent of the population (see Figure 1.4).

Figure 1.5 presents the population growth and expected growth for a hundred-year period, 1950 to 2050, in different age categories. As was mentioned above, the total population will increase to almost 450 million people. It is interesting to see the growth since 1990 in the age groups sixty-five years and

FIGURE 1.4: Projected population percentage by race, 2010 to 2050, in the United States

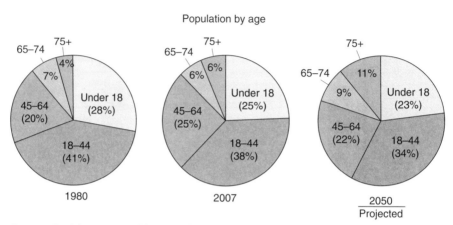

Source: CDC/NCHS, *Health, United States, 2009*, Figure 1B. Data from the U.S. Census Bureau.

FIGURE 1.5: Population growth in the United States, 2010 to 2050

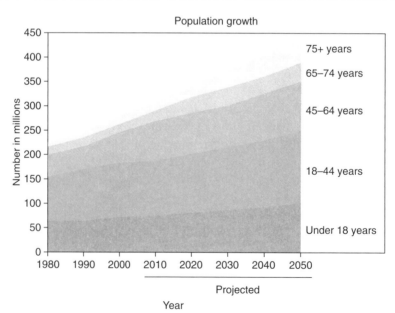

Source: CDC/NCHS, *Health, United States, 2009*, Figure 1A. Data from the U.S. Census Bureau.

older and seventy-five years and older. These two age groups are contributing to the overall increase in the population because people are living longer.

Population Characteristics

Other aspects of the U.S. population need to be presented to fully understand the dynamics and characteristics. The *life expectancy* of the population is an important concern of public health. Life expectancy indicates the health of the country and the quality of life of the population. Figure 1.6 presents the projected life expectancy in the United States by sex, from 2010 to 2050.

The projected life expectancy is expected to increase for both men and women over the next forty years. The projected increase will be greater for women than for men. By the year 2050, the gap between men and women will narrow, with women expected to live 4.6 years longer than men.

Figure 1.7 presents the projected life expectancy according to race and gender, at birth and after a person has reached sixty-five years of age. This shows how long someone is expected to live in total years from birth and how much longer someone should live past age sixty-five. White women have the highest life expectancy, closely followed by black women, from birth and at age sixty-five.

FIGURE 1.6: Projected life expectancy in years by sex, United States, 2010 to 2050

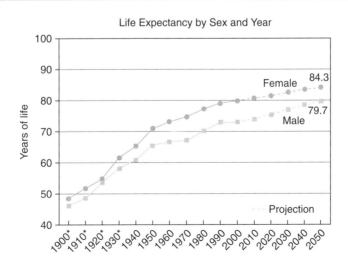

Life Expectancy by Sex and Year

FIGURE 1.7: Life expectancy from birth and at age 65 years by race and gender, United States, 1970 to 2005

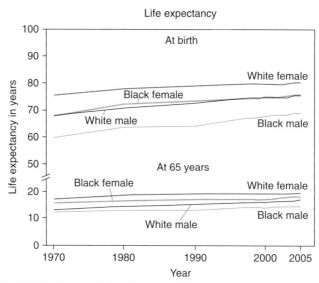

Source: CDC/NCHS, *Health, United States, 2009,* Figure 16. Data from the National Vital Statistics System.

The health of infants and newborns is an indicator of the overall health status of a population. The United States is seen as a world leader in many things, including health care services. However, the United States has a higher death rate among infants and newborns than many other industrialized countries. This will be discussed in more detail in Chapter Five.

On a positive note, the death rates from infants and newborns have drastically decreased in recent times. Figure 1.8 shows infant mortality, neonatal, and postneonatal mortality rates from 1950 to 2006. Each rate has decreased greatly during the fifty-four-year period. For example, the infant mortality rate (the measurement of the number of deaths before age one year) decreased from almost 30 deaths per 1,000 live births in 1950 to less than 10 deaths in 2006. This is an indication that social, medical, and educational interventions have been successful in reducing deaths of infants and newborns. Again this shows how epidemiology, in conjunction with public health programs, has made our lives better.

FIGURE 1.8: Death rates of infants and newborns,
United States, 1950 to 2005

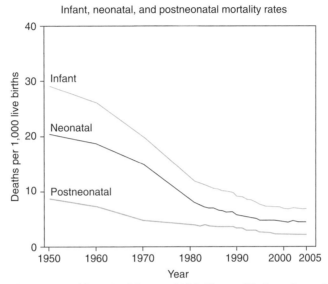

Infant, neonatal, and postneonatal mortality rates

Source: CDC/NCHS, *Health, United States, 2009*, Figure 17. Data from the National Vital Statistics System.

Health Costs

It is interesting to note how much it costs for our health care, including public health services, each year in the United States. In 2007 the total health care costs were $1.9 trillion. Figure 1.9 shows how this money was spent for health care services and what were the sources of funding.

Looking at where the money is spent, the majority goes to hospitals and physicians. Other areas of spending are nursing home care and prescription drugs. It is also clear that most of the money for health care services comes from insurance, both private and federally funded. Some funds come from state and local programs, with the remainder paid by people who use the services.

With such a large health care industry and an equally large health insurance industry, it seems that all Americans should receive needed care. But this is not the case. Figure 1.10 shows the percentage of health insurance coverage for people younger than sixty-five years in the United States (Americans sixty-five

FIGURE 1.9: Funding health care in the United States

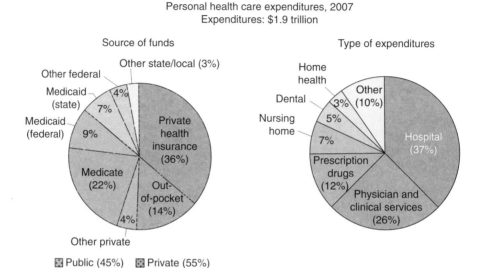

Personal health care expenditures, 2007
Expenditures: $1.9 trillion

Source of funds

Type of expenditures

Other state/local (3%)
Other federal
Medicaid (state) 4%
7%
Medicaid (federal) 9%
Private health insurance (36%)
Medicate (22%)
Out-of-pocket (14%)
4%
Other private

Home health
Dental 3%
Other (10%)
Nursing home 5%
7%
Prescription drugs (12%)
Hospital (37%)
Physician and clinical services (26%)

Public (45%)   Private (55%)

Source: CDC/NCHS, *Health, United States, 2009*, Figure 21. Data from the Centers for Medicare & Medicaid Services.

FIGURE 1.10: Health insurance coverage among people younger than 65 years

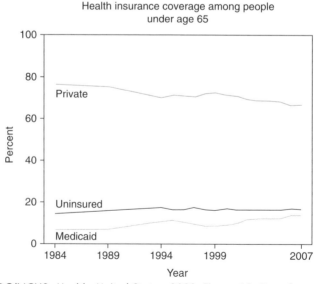

Health insurance coverage among people under age 65

Private

Uninsured

Medicaid

Percent

Year

Source: CDC/NCHS, *Health, United States, 2009*, Figure 19. Data from the National Health Interview Survey.

years and older are eligible to receive Medicare benefits). The percentage of Americans who are uninsured has increased nearly 20 percent in the past twenty-five years. It is important to remember that the total population in the United States has significantly increased since 1984, so the number of uninsured Americans has drastically increased as well.

Global Health Threats

Today, epidemiology and public health face many challenges such as chronic diseases, West Nile virus, AIDS, and the worry over pandemic flu. As the world is getting progressively smaller with rapid methods to travel, global health threats are occurring everywhere, including in the United States. According to the World Health Organization (WHO), by the year 2030, chronic and noncommunicable diseases will cause more than 75 percent of all deaths. Today 12 percent of all deaths worldwide are caused by heart disease whereas 3.5 percent of deaths are a result of HIV/AIDS. By 2030, more than 14 percent of deaths will be caused by heart disease, with HIV/AIDS deaths decreasing to 1.9 percent. Diseases and conditions that are receiving attention globally today include infant mortality, neonatal mortality, HIV/AIDS, malaria, effects of tobacco use, breast cancer, and disease outbreaks in developing countries.

When we talk about global health threats, we usually discuss possible pandemics of infectious diseases. However, our attention should shift to chronic and non-communicable diseases and conditions. Although infectious diseases are an immediate worry, more people today die from chronic diseases. The worry of infectious diseases is rooted in the unknown and unexpected effects of pandemics. The science of epidemiology can help us to sort real threats from unwarranted concerns.

Summary

In this chapter we introduced the science known as epidemiology and its role in public health. The ways in which our everyday lives are touched, whether we know it or not, by epidemiology and public health was described. In addition, examples of how public health and epidemiology have positively affected people's lives were presented. The emphasis from infectious disease to chronic and infectious diseases was discussed.

Key Terms

Causal factors, 4   Public health, 9

Life expectancy, 13   Social epidemiology, 10

Chapter Exercise

1. Define epidemiology.
2. Compare and contrast medicine and public health.
3. Discuss in some detail one of the public health accomplishments that was mentioned in the chapter.

Chapter Review

1. Epidemiology has been defined as the
   a. study of epidemic diseases.
   b. study of clinical diseases.
   c. study of the distribution and determinants of disease in human populations.
   d. the basic service of health education.
2. Epidemiology is a branch of public health. True or False?
3. The leading cause of death in the United States is
   a. cancer.
   b. heart disease.
   c. automobile accidents.
   d. stroke.
4. The U.S. population is expected to increase for all races between 2010 and 2050. True or False?
5. The projected life expectancy in the United States in the year 2005 is greater for blacks than for all other races. True or False?
6. Neonatal mortality rates have increased from 1950 to 2004. True or False
7. The number of Americans who are uninsured has stayed the same since 1964. True or False?
8. Most money spent on health care goes for hospital and physician services. True or False?

WHY EPIDEMIOLOGY? 19

9. In 2005 the federal government provided most of the funds for health care services in the United States. True or False?
10. By the year 2050, the percentage of whites in the United States will
    a. increase.
    b. remain the same.
    c. decrease.
    d. cannot be determined

CHAPTER 2

HISTORY OF EPIDEMIOLOGY

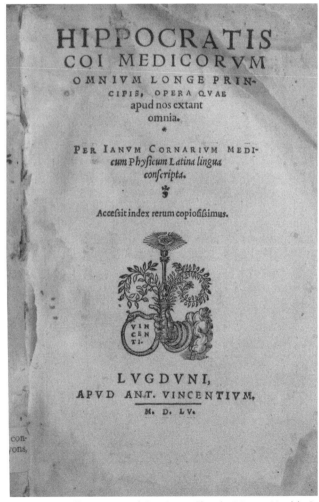

HIPPOCRATIS
COI MEDICORVM
OMNIVM LONGE PRIN-
CIPIS, OPERA QVAE
apud nos extant
omnia.

PER IANVM CORNARIVM MEDI-
cum Phyficum Latina lingua
confcripta.

Accefsit index rerum copiofifsimus.

LVGDVNI,
APVD ANT. VINCENTIVM,
M. D. LV.

Courtesy of Historical Collections and Services, Claude Moore Health Sciences
Library, University of Virginia, Charlottesville.

LEARNING OBJECTIVES

On completing this chapter, you should be able to

Discuss the history of epidemiology
Describe the contributions of people in history
Describe the uses of epidemiology
Describe examples of how epidemiology has been used to study disease prevention

Historical Perspectives

Prehistoric Times

From the time that humans first began to inhabit the earth, health and disease has been a part of life. As the earth's population continued to grow and expand its geographical reach, many diseases began to occur. The notion of "survival of the fittest" can be extended to assume that early humans acquired over time an understanding of the relationship between the environment and health. It is reasonable to think the prehistoric people were aware of their environment and took precautions. In addition to avoiding natural predators, prehistoric people were careful about the foods they ate and water they drank. Foods and water sources that made them sick or die were no longer consumed. As this knowledge was passed along to others in the population, the seeds of epidemiology were planted. As humans continued to inhabit the earth and as the population increased and spread out geographically, this knowledge became more and more important. For example, passing on information about obtaining and using animal hides and furs as protective clothing helped to increase survival in a predatory world.

Greeks

Basic epidemiological methods were mentioned in the Bible. In the book of Numbers, Moses conducted the first recorded census. However, the Greeks continued the development of epidemiology into a scientific discipline. Hippocrates, who lived from 460 to 377 BC, wrote the classic work "On Airs, Waters, and Places" as an explanation of why epidemics and plagues happened. Hippocrates presented evidence suggesting that environmental and behavioral factors could be associated with disease. His work began what is referred to today as environmental epidemiology. Hippocrates provided accurate descriptions of the diseases tetanus, typhus, and phthisis.[1] For his work, which is the first time scientific methods were used to study disease, Hippocrates is considered the father of epidemiology and the world's first epidemiologist.[2]

Egyptians

The ancient Egyptians are known for their medical advances, including surgeries to treat illness. They did not have an organized public health system, but they did discover and practice several public health interventions. First, Egyptians had a full understanding of cleanliness and its effect on health. They used baths and toilets. For religious reasons, personal cleanliness and physical appearance were important.

Egyptians practiced disease prevention. Egyptian men and women wore eye makeup because they believed that this would protect their eyes from diseases. They used mosquito nets at night to protect themselves from diseases transmitted by insects. It was common for Egyptians to use amulets, charms, and spells to protect themselves and others from diseases. Diet and nutrition were recognized as having a relationship with health. An ancient Egyptian's diet was typically balanced, with cereals, fruit, and fish as major food choices. Milk, milk products, seeds, and oil were not major foods in their diets.

History tells us the Egyptian priests served as religious leaders and healers. They frequently cast spells to prevent disease, treated people and animals, and may have had knowledge about links between diseased animals and diseased people. It is thought that Egyptian priests may have had the ability to prevent epidemics by inspecting animals that were used for religious sacrifices.[3] Diseases that originate with animals and are spread to humans are called zoonoses, or zoonotic diseases. Today's examples of zoonotic diseases include West Nile virus, severe acute respiratory syndrome (SARS), mad cow disease, and bird flu and swine flu.

Romans

Medicine and public health in ancient Rome were greatly influenced by the Greeks, especially after Greece became a Roman province. The Romans placed a great deal of importance on public health because they believed that cleanliness was linked to good health. They focused on the prevention of diseases and established a public health system that was seen in all parts of the Roman Empire. In fact, the Romans felt that prevention was more important than treatment of diseases. The Roman public health system benefited all people in the empire, not only the rich.

The Romans paid attention to the environment and knew where to build their houses and other buildings. Cities were built along waterways or areas with natural springs. Houses were built with toilets. They recognized that disease was more prevalent in areas near swamps and marshes. With this knowledge, Romans drained marshes to eliminate areas that bred disease-carrying mosquitos. This shows that the Romans had an appreciation for environmental epidemiology, as did the Greeks.

The Romans emphasized that keeping physically fit was a key to staying healthy. Because the Roman Empire was dependent on an imposing army, the health of soldiers was of greatest importance. Soldiers were always provided clean water. Camps were never located near swamps, and swamp water was never consumed. Soldiers were encouraged to stay physically fit and were moved around often to decrease exposure to diseases prevalent in particular places.

The Romans were committed to providing clean water to all citizens. Because the Romans were technically advanced, they built an elaborate aqueduct system to provide clean water. They built sewers to remove sewage, as well as public toilets in cities. Personal hygiene was important, and public baths were constructed throughout the Roman Empire. Both rich and poor Romans used these public baths.[4]

Fifteenth to Seventeenth Centuries

Before the Middle Ages, public health and epidemiology were used to respond to disease. This response was based on preventive measures, as discussed above. During the Middle Ages, the interest of epidemiology shifted from environmental factors to understanding the specific cause of disease. For example, what substance in the drinking water causes illness, or what was in a mosquito bite that resulted in disease?

The first person to address these questions was Girolamo Fracastorius, who lived from 1478 to 1553. He first proposed what is now known as germ theory.[5] He studied epidemics and was the first to make a science-backed statement of the nature of contagion, infection, disease germs, and modes of transmission. He identified ways in which infections can be transmitted. He discovered that infection was transmitted by direct contact, through droplet spread, from contaminated clothing, and through the air. Several hundred years later, Louis Pasteur would prove his theories accurate.

Natural and *Political*

OBSERVATIONS

Mentioned in a following INDEX,

and made upon the

Bills of Mortality.

By *JOHN GRAUNT,*

Citizen of

LONDON.

With reference to the *Government, Religion, Trade, Growth, Ayre, Diseases,* and the several Changes of the said CITY.

—— *Non, me ut miretur Turba, laboro, Contentus paucis Lectoribus* ——

LONDON,

Printed by *Tho: Roycroft,* for *John Martin, James Allestry,* and *Tho: Dicas,* at the Sign of the Bell in St. *Paul's* Church-yard, MDCLXII.

Observational epidemiology, which is based on observing the relationship between disease and disease-causing factors, began as a science in the 1600s due to the work of John Graunt, who lived from 1620 to 1674. Graunt was a statistician who used empirical observations of causes of death and compiled the first mortality tables, using England's bills of mortality, which were records of deaths. Today we use death certificates. Graunt is called the father of *demography*, which is the statistical study of human populations according to size and density, distribution, and vital statistics (births, marriages, deaths, and so forth). He was the first to classify and categorize deaths according to the cause and calculated death rates by these categories.[6] His contribution was such that his work is referred to as the starting point of modern epidemiology.

Another seventeenth-century epidemiologist was Thomas Sydenham, who is called the English Hippocrates.[7] Sydenham reemphasized the theories of Hippocrates and expanded them for use in the seventeenth century. He was the first to describe the clinical manifestations of Bell's palsy, a condition that causes the facial muscles to weaken or become paralyzed. Like Hippocrates, he used scientific observations of health and wove them into the core fabric of modern epidemiology.

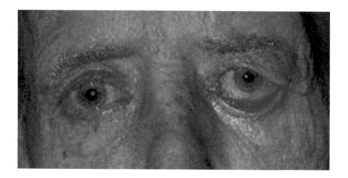

Eighteenth Century

James Lind (1716–1794), a Scottish surgery apprentice, was the first known clinical epidemiologist. As a pioneer of naval hygiene, he worked as surgeon's mate and sailed for many years around the world. He performed experiments in an attempt to determine the cause of scurvy. Scurvy, which causes loose teeth, bleeding gums, and hemorrhages, affected sailors. Lind adjusted their diets by adding foods such as cider, garlic, mustard, horseradish, vinegar, oranges, and lemons. He noted that the sailors who ate oranges and lemons recovered from the effects of scurvy, proving Lind's theory that citrus fruits were the best treatment for the disease. Today we know that scurvy is caused by a vitamin C deficiency. Later in his life, Lind contributed to the knowledge of typhus fever on ships and chronicled diseases.

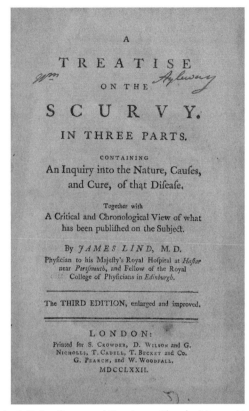

Courtesy of Historical Collections and Services, Claude Moore Health Sciences Library, University of Virginia, Charlottesville.

Nineteenth Century

The second recognized clinical epidemiologist was Pierre Charles Alexandre Louis (1787–1872). Louis was a French physician who became known for his research on tuberculosis, typhoid fever, and the use of bloodletting for the treatment of pneumonia. He was the first to collect data from groups of patients to gain information about a disease. He used this information to describe the natural history and clinical presentation of a disease. He found that bloodletting, a common treatment at the time, was ineffective against pneumonia and fevers.

William Farr (1807–1883) established a national system for recording causes of death in England.[8] This standard classification system was the beginning of disease and death cataloguing, which today is done by the International

Classification of Diseases and Related Conditions. Farr was involved in the first modern census, which was used to collect specific information on diseases and conditions (blindness and deafness), and he also invented the *standardized mortality rate,* which is a measure of the number of deaths in a population per unit of time: for example, the number of deaths per 1,000 individuals per year.

John Snow (1813–1858) made the greatest contribution to epidemiology during the nineteenth century. Snow used epidemiological principles to study outbreaks of cholera in London in the 1850s.[9] He showed how scientific evidence can be used to support theories, hypotheses, and analytical investigations. He identified the source of the infectious agent, which was contaminated water, and how the cholera outbreak started and spread throughout London.[10] His work has been described as a brilliant use of descriptive and quantitative epidemiological principles.[11]

Twentieth Century

As the twentieth century began, epidemiology was involved with infectious and communicable diseases. In 1900 the leading cause of death was pneumonia and influenza, followed closely by tuberculosis. Other leading causes of death in 1900 were diarrhea, heart disease, and nephritis. As the twentieth century progressed, chronic diseases became more pronounced as causes of death. In 1930 heart disease became the leading cause of death, as it is today. The emergence of chronic diseases as the leading health concern continued through the 1940s and 1950s, with infectious diseases becoming less of a concern. The difference between the death rates of chronic and infectious diseases was widening as the twentieth century moved along. By the end of the twentieth century, the only infectious diseases remaining in the top ten of leading causes of death were pneumonia and influenza.

With the shifting of disease impact from infectious and communicable to those chronic in nature, epidemiology continued to evolve with a focus on individual diseases and conditions. New ways to study diseases were developed, beginning in the 1930s. Epidemiologists began to study tobacco uses and its long-term health effects. In the 1960s, the Surgeon General first reported on the relationship between smoking and death from coronary artery disease. The report did not identify a causal relationship, but it did state an association between cigarette smoking and many cardiovascular diseases.[12] Hospital-based cohort studies on cigarette smoking began in 1950.[13] Cohort studies follow the same group of people through a period of time. Well-known cohort studies include the Framingham Heart Study and the Bogalusa Heart Study. The Framingham and Bogalusa studies are presented later in this chapter.

Twenty-First Century

In the twenty-first century, epidemiology expanded its focus to health status, health-related quality of life, and burden of disease. In addition, the events of September 11, 2001, resulted in epidemiology gaining a role in bioterrorism preparedness and management of health care services. The infectious and communicable disease focus of epidemiology has also become more prominent recently (as it was in the early twentieth century) owing to the significant number of emerging infectious diseases (including AIDS, bird flu, SARS, and H1N1 flu). It is expected that this focus will diminish over the next several years and that chronic and non-communicable diseases will be at the forefront of epidemiology and public health in our future.

Uses of Epidemiology

Since its beginnings, epidemiology has looked for ways to describe health and disease and factors that affect health and disease. During its development, epidemiology evolved into a science that once only observed health and disease to one that also used experimental methods. Epidemiology today has expanded to include the study of injuries, chronic and infectious diseases, environmental and occupational conditions that affect health, and bioterrorism.

In its evolution, epidemiology has been linked with medicine. This medical association has been seen as epidemiology assisting in the following:

1. determining etiological or causal factors of diseases;

2. describing factors that are associated with adverse conditions;

3. describing the distribution of a disease in a community;

4. predicting disease occurrence, impact, and distribution in a community;

5. estimating a person's chance of suffering from diseases;

6. evaluating preventive, therapeutic, and intervention activities;

7. measuring efficacy of health measures;

8. studying historical disease trends; (9) identifying disease syndromes;

9. planning for current health care needs; and

10. predicting future health care needs.

Community diagnosis is important, and facts about the health of a community can be described using epidemiology. Epidemiological information shows how severe a disease is and the number of people affected by the disease. By using specific epidemiological measurements, we can compare health problems with other instances of the same population at other times or in other communities. The description of the distribution of health in different segments of the population is helpful in understanding the full impact of a health problem.

Another aspect of community diagnosis is estimating a person's risk (or chance) of getting a disease. Understanding the future disease possibilities is as important as knowing how much disease is in the community today. Many epidemiological methods are used to predict the chance that someone will get a disease. These include specific epidemiological measures, known as *rates*, and epidemiological ratios, known as *risk ratios*. The predictive nature of these epidemiological measurements and methods is useful in trying to understand the future effects of diseases in a community and what will be needed to fight these diseases.

Another major use of epidemiology is in preventing disease. In fact, prevention can be reviewed in three categories. First is *primary prevention*, which is useful in control of the distribution, frequency, and severity of diseases. Primary prevention is focused on preventing new cases of a disease. This happens by removing factors that cause changes that result in a disease developing. Health education is an example of a primary prevention activity. Other examples are purification of water supplies, immunization, protection from occupational hazards by wearing hard hats, and wearing seat belts.

The second category, known as *secondary prevention,* is involved with stopping diseases after they have begun. Secondary prevention involves screening, early disease detection, and early treatment of disease. The final category is called *tertiary prevention,* and its aim is to improve health and survival of people who have diseases that cannot be cured. Rehabilitation activities that stop the progression of a disease or disability are examples of tertiary prevention.

Examples of Cohort Studies

The Framingham Heart Study

Diseases of the heart have been the leading cause of death in the United States since the 1930s. To study heart disease, the Framingham Heart Study was begun in 1948 with the purpose of identifying the contributors to coronary heart disease. The Framingham Heart Study was designed to study large groups of people (called cohorts) over a long period of time. The people studied had no heart disease at the beginning of the study, and they were observed over many years. The study started with more than five thousand people (men and women) between the ages of thirty and sixty-two years, all residents of Framingham, Massachusetts. Beginning in 1948, after physical examinations and lifestyle interviews, the people went through medical examinations every two years. The Framingham Heart Study continues today with the children and grandchildren of the original five thousand people.[14]

The Framingham Heart Study has resulted in identifying factors that put people at high risk for developing heart disease. These factors include high blood pressure, high cholesterol levels, smoking, obesity, diabetes, and physical inactivity. Today the Framingham Heart Study is researching how genetics plays a part in the development of heart disease.[15]

The Bogalusa Heart Study

The Bogalusa Heart Study is a cohort study of heart disease in white and African American children and adolescents.[16] The Bogalusa Heart Study began in 1973 with the intention of studying the early natural history of cardiovascular disease, which appears in older ages as hypertension and atherosclerosis. To date, more than sixteen thousand people, ages birth to forty-five years, have participated in the study. Subjects have been categorized into pediatric (ages three to twenty) and adult (ages twenty to forty-five) groups. Questionnaires are administered to determine educational status, occupation, smoking and family medical histories, and levels of physical activities. Clinical examinations include blood pressure, lipid blood levels, and other blood tests.

The Bogalusa Heart Study has uncovered many significant findings. It has become obvious that cardiovascular disease begins in children, with clinical evidence seen as early as five years of age. Cardiovascular disease risk factors can be identified at early ages, and through public health programs, these risk factors can be reduced or eliminated. The level and effect of risk factors vary at different ages. Other findings show that African Americans have more severe forms of hypertension than whites. Environmental factors place a major role in the development of cardiovascular disease. These include diet, exercise, and smoking.[17]

Summary

In this chapter we presented the history of epidemiology and public health from ancient times to the present. The contributions of the Greeks, Egyptians. and Romans were highlighted. The developments of public health and epidemiology and the contributors, from the fifteenth to the twenty-first century were described.

The uses of epidemiology, which have a positive influence on everyday life today, were explained in detail.

Key Terms

Demography, 25

Observational epidemiology, 25

Primary prevention, 30

Secondary prevention, 30

Tertiary prevention, 30

Standardized mortality rate, 28

Zoonotic diseases, 23

Chapter Exercises

1. Describe five uses of epidemiology and give examples.
2. Define the three categories of prevention.
3. Discuss the contributions of the Egyptians and Romans to epidemiology and public health.

Chapter Review

1. The father of epidemiology is considered to be the Greek, Aristotle. True or False?
2. Early Egyptians appeared to understand the importance of proper nutrition. True or False?
3. The first ancient people to use public sanitation on a large scale were the
   a. Greeks.
   b. Romans.
   c. Egyptians.
   d. seventeenth-century Europeans.
4. The creator of the germ theory was
   a. Graunt.
   b. Lister.
   c. Fracastorius.
   d. Pasteur.
5. The founder of observational epidemiology was
   a. Graunt.
   b. Lister.

c. Fracastorius.

d. Pasteur.

6. The English Hippocrates was John Gruant. True or False?

7. The first clinical epidemiologist was

a. James Lind.

b. Louis Pasteur.

c. John Graunt.

d. Hippocrates.

8. John Snow used epidemiological principles to study cholera outbreaks in London. True or False?

9. Before 1910, the leading cause of death in the United States was

a. pneumonia.

b. tuberculosis.

c. heart disease.

d. malnutrition.

10. Epidemiology is used in

a. estimating a person's chance of getting a disease.

b. community diagnosis of the distribution of a disease.

c. determining etiology of a disease.

d. all of the above.

e. none of the above.

HEALTH AND DISEASE

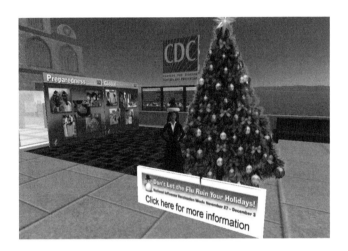

LEARNING OBJECTIVES

On completing this chapter, you will be able to

Discuss what is meant by health
Discuss what is meant by disease
Describe the distinction between health and disease
Describe the natural history of disease
Discuss the general concept of causal relationships

Definitions

Health is something that seems easy to identify and measure. We can take our temperature to see if we have a fever. We can get blood tests to determine disease. But what about quality of life? How is it measured? In this chapter, we will discuss what is meant by health and the notion of health-related quality of life. Should more attention be given to how health and disease affect our everyday life, and not on measuring health test results? In this chapter, we will explore this question, but first, let's define health and disease.

Health

The World Health Organization defines *health* as a state of complete physical, mental, and social well-being and not merely the absence of disease or infirmity.[1] This definition was ratified during the first World Health Assembly and has not been changed since 1948. In 2000 Pope John Paul II offered a more comprehensive definition of health as "A dynamic tension towards physical, mental, social, and spiritual harmony, and not only the absence of illness, which gives man the ability to fulfill the mission which has been entrusted to him."[2]

Health has two aspects that influence it. The first is *physical health*, which is often referred to as physical fitness. Physical health is dependent on proper nutrition, exercise, and other healthy life behaviors. The other aspect of health is mental health. *Mental health* is defined as "A state of emotional and psychological well-being in which an individual is able to use his or her cognitive and emotional capabilities, function in society, and meet the ordinary demands of everyday life" (*Merriam-Webster Online Dictionary*, http://www.merriam-webster.com/dictionary/mentalhealth, 2008). Mental health has a significant role in overall health and is considered emotional and psychological well-being.

There are four major determinants of health: our biological makeup, the environment, our lifestyle, and the availability and our use of health care services.[3] To a certain extent, we can change or improve our biological makeup, and we can affect the influence of the other three health determinants. For example, an environmental factor that affects health is water quality. Public health initiatives work to provide us a clean and safe water supply. We can improve our lifestyle with a proper diet, nutrition, and exercise. Regular physical exercise is important in the prevention of cancer, obesity, and back pain and is essential for staying physically fit.

Another aspect of lifestyle that can affect our health is stress. Stress negatively influences health by weakening our immune system. Exercise can improve physical fitness and boost the immune system to counterbalance the effects of stress. Relaxation techniques are also helpful in reducing stress as is positive thinking. Improvement of problem-solving and time-management skills can reduce stress and improve health.

Disease

Disease is an abnormal condition of an organism that impairs bodily functions associated with specific symptoms and signs. It is "a pathological condition of a part, organ, or system of an organism resulting from various causes, such as infection, genetic defect, or environmental stress, and characterized by an identifiable group of signs or symptoms" (*American Heritage Dictionary*, 4th edition).

Distinction Between Health and Disease

Sometimes disease is defined more broadly as the absence of health. This is not always accurate because a person with a disease may lead a life that follows the definition of health. For example, someone with controlled diabetes has a disease but may exhibit optimal well-being and lead a productive life. The presence of disease doesn't mean that someone is ill. Illness involves a subjective (mental) component. In fact, someone may feel ill but not have a disease. Figure 3.1 presents a matrix of illness and disease. This matrix shows that people may feel ill both when they have and do not have a disease.

FIGURE 3.1: Illness-disease matrix

DISEASE	ILLNESS IS PRESENT	ILLNESS IS ABSENT
DISEASE IS PRESENT	Disease Is Present and Person Feels Ill	Disease Is Present but the Person Feels Well
DISEASE IS ABSENT	Disease Is Absent but Person Feels Ill	Disease Is Absent and Person Feels Well

Because medical care providers usually focus their attention on disease, health is not typically measured directly. However, descriptive disease measurement is used as an indication of health status. If descriptive data indicate a lack of or a relatively low level of disease, then the level of health is considered to be high.

Quality of Life

Quality of life (QoL) is a measurement that represents an overall feeling of well-being. QoL is difficult to understand and measure because it is a complex and subjective concept, with no common measurement. *Health-related quality of life* (HRQL) is a measurement of the general QoL that affects overall health. HRQL measures both physical and mental health[4] or a person's physical and mental self-perceptions of his or her health.[5] HRQL is gaining popularity as a measure of perceived physical and mental health and function and as an indicator of health resources needed for a population.[6]

HRQL measurement can be classified into two categories: generic health and disease-specific measures. HRQL measurements are usually self-administered questionnaires. In public health, these are used to measure a person's perceived physical and mental health over a period of time. For example, HRQL is used to measure the effects of chronic illness, such as cancer, and how it affects a person's day-to-day life. HRQL can be tracked in different populations to determine which subgroups are adversely affected by perceptions of physical and mental health. The Centers for Disease Control and Prevention has determined the following:

- people in the United States feel unhealthy (physically or mentally) about six days per month,

- people in the United States feel "healthy and full of energy" about nineteen days per month,

- almost one third of the people in the United States suffer from some mental or emotional problem every month,

- people aged eighteen to twenty-four years most frequently suffer mental health distress,

- older people experience the most activity limitation, and

- people with chronic diseases report high levels of unhealthy days.[7]

Disease Progression

Natural History of Disease

The *natural history of a disease* is the description of the progression of a disease from the first sign or manifestation of the disease until recovery or death. It is important to know about the natural history of a disease to help prevent, treat, and control a disease, and as such, it is one of the major parts of descriptive epidemiology. *Descriptive epidemiology* involves studying the amount of disease that is occurring in a population and describing this according to characteristics and traits of the people in the population. These characteristics and traits include age, race, sex, where people live, and when disease is occurring.

The natural history of a disease is what would occur if there were no medical treatment. Because people usually receive some form of treatment for diseases, it may be helpful to think of the natural history as the clinical course. The *clinical course of a disease* is what happens when people are being treated for the disease. The clinical course can be described by five stages. The first is the stage in which a person does not have a disease, but they may be susceptible to it. The second stage is when a person has a disease, but it is not causing any symptoms and it is too early to detect the disease. During this stage the person is not receiving treatment. The third stage also does not cause any symptoms, but screening tests will detect it. The fourth stage is when diagnosis usually takes place. In this stage symptoms are obvious, and it is during this time that people usually seek treatment. The final stage is when the disease outcomes occur, that is, death or recovery.

If we can understand the natural history of disease, then we can begin to determine the course of a disease and whether someone will recover from the effects of a disease, which is called the prognosis. *Prognosis* of a disease is predicting the future symptoms and outcomes of a disease.[8] Prognosis describes what is frequently seen with a disease. Prognostic factors and predisposing conditions are descriptive in terms of disease outcomes, including disability and death. Throughout the book, we will discuss the natural history of two diseases, type 2 diabetes and AIDS.

Type 2 diabetes is also called adult-onset or non-insulin-dependent diabetes. In early stages, it does not cause symptoms. Its early development is unknown to the person with diabetes. During its progression, to a point that the person begins to have health problems, type 2 diabetes is seen as a mild hyperglycemia. *Hyperglycemia* has several symptoms, including high levels of blood sugar (called glucose), high levels of sugar in the urine, frequent urination, and increased thirst. High blood glucose levels happen when the body does not have enough insulin or the insulin cannot be used by the body (this is called insulin resistance). *Insulin* is a hormone that is secreted by the body to reduce high levels of glucose in the blood. When a person is found to have mild hyperglycemia, he or she is at risk for the development of diabetes, and early treatment can begin. This treatment involves patient education, diet and nutrition changes, exercise, and medications. It is estimated that more than 22 million people in the United States have mild hyperglycemia.[9] When type 2 diabetes progresses, medical treatment becomes necessary.

Type 2 diabetes causes metabolic problems, which result in the adverse effects of the disease. No one knows what causes type 2 diabetes, but it is suspected that genetics may play a role in its development. Type 2 diabetes is seen most frequently in families and specific racial and ethnic groups, including Hispanics, African Americans, Pacific Islanders, and American Indians. Besides genetics, many other factors are associated with type 2 diabetes, including age, obesity, poor diet and nutrition, and lack of physical exercise and activity. Obesity plays a large role in the development of type 2 diabetes because obese people typically have insulin resistance. Knowing its natural history, the treatment of type 2 diabetes should begin early so the effects of the disease can be minimized. Identifying and treating people with mild hyperglycemia reduces the number who go on to develop type 2 diabetes. Early treatment of those who do develop type 2 diabetes reduces the adverse effects of the disease and lessens the bad effects.

Type 2 diabetes can be prevented by proper diet, exercise, and weight loss in obese people. These factors can help to prevent type 2 diabetes whether they are used alone or in combination. A more profound improvement results if these factors are implemented at the same time. The Malmo Feasibility Study showed that weight loss and improved physical fitness each improved health and prevented the development of type 2 diabetes. The study also showed that when weight loss and an improved physical fitness program were used together, the improvement in health was doubled.[10] Many medications are available for the treatment of type 2 diabetes, but none of these assist in its prevention. The medications have been successful in improving insulin resistance for short periods of time, but this improvement is not permanent.[11]

As was mentioned in Chapter One, AIDS is the final stage of HIV infection. Before discussing the natural of history of AIDS, let's discuss the factors that cause AIDS. They are predisposing, starting, and maintenance factors. Today it is known that the factors for AIDS are different depending on whether you are in an underdeveloped or a developed country. An *underdeveloped country* is one that, when compared with others, has a low per capita income because of the absence of industrialization and infrastructure. A country's gross national product is also used for classification.

In developed countries (which include the United States), the predisposing factors for AIDS usually include illicit drug use, blood transfusions, and unprotected sexual activity. Other factors, such as stress, anxiety, and depression, contribute to weakening the immune system, which increases the risk of AIDS.[12,13] In underdeveloped countries, the most important predisposing factor is poor nutrition. The absence of proper nutrition is a lifelong struggle, starting as a fetus and ending at death.[14] Other factors include infections caused by less-than-adequate sanitation, mental stress, antibiotic usage, and chemical pollution.[15,16]

AIDS starting factors have the same pattern as predisposing factors. In developed countries, drug usage is the most significant starting factor. The effects of environmental pollution and other viral and bacterial infection (syphilis) also can be starting factors.[17] The most common AIDS starting factor in underdeveloped countries is a new infection (or parasitosis) in a previously malnourished and debilitated person.[18] In fact, a specific nutritional deficiency can be a starting factor.[19] Stress and alcohol, acting alone or together, also have been shown to be starting factors for AIDS.[20]

Maintenance factors continue and may worsen the progression of AIDS and are the same as predisposing and starting factors in both developed and underdeveloped countries. The only uniqueness is when the factors are influencing the natural history of AIDS. The key manifestation of AIDS is a deficiency in the immune system. This immunodeficiency is caused by the degeneration of immune cells.[21,22] In AIDS, three main functions of the immune system are all adversely affected: defense, homeostasis, and surveillance.

It is important to understand whether a known factor is indeed a risk factor. A set of criteria exists that can be used to decide whether a factor affects the risk of getting a disease. The criteria are the temporal relationship between the cause and effect, strength of the association, the dose-response relationship, reversible associations, consistency, plausibility, specificity, and analogy.[23]

AIDS is associated with, and is caused by, the human immunosuppressive virus, known as HIV. As the final stage of HIV infection, all people who have AIDS also have HIV infection. Where did HIV come from, and how long has it been affecting people? The HIV virus is similar to a simian virus found in monkeys and baboons. In Africa monkeys are used as pets and a food source. In fact, the earliest known case of HIV infection occurred in the Congo in 1959. In the United States, the first known case of AIDS was in 1952, with the first recorded case occurring in 1981.

WHAT IS WEST NILE VIRUS?

West Nile virus (WNV) is a potentially serious illness, considered as a seasonal epidemic in North America, that begins in the summer and lasts into the fall.

Symptoms of WNV

- About 1 in 150 people infected with WNV will develop severe illness. Symptoms include high fever, headache, neck stiffness, stupor, disorientation, coma, tremors, convulsions, muscle weakness, vision loss, numbness, and paralysis. Symptoms may be seen for several weeks, and neurological effects may be permanent.

- As many as 20 percent of the people who become infected have milder symptoms, including fever, headache and body aches, nausea, vomiting, and sometimes swollen lymph glands or a skin rash on the chest, stomach, and back. Symptoms can last from a few days to several weeks.

- Approximately 80 percent of people (about four out of five) who are infected with WNV will not have any symptoms.

Source: Centers for Disease Control and Prevention, http://www.cdc.gov/ncidod/dvbid/westnile/wnv_factsheet.htm.

Disease Transmission

Disease can be transmitted in many ways. Infectious diseases are transmitted by direct and indirect ways. With respect to infectious disease, the following terms must be understood. A reservoir is a person, animal, insect, plant, or substance in which the infectious agent usually lives and multiples. A host is any susceptible person.

Direct transmission of a disease is caused by coughing and sneezing and through kissing and sexual intercourse. Sexually transmitted diseases (STDs) are infections that occur because of direct transmission. Examples of STDs include venereal diseases, chlamydial infections, trichomonal infections, herpes, and AIDS.

Indirect ways that diseases are transmitted include vehicle-borne, vector-borne, and airborne transmission. *Vehicle-borne transmission* happens when diseases are transmitted by contaminated food and water. Other examples of vehicle-borne transmission include contaminated inanimate materials or objects (called fomites) such as toys, handkerchiefs, soiled clothes, bedding, cooking or eating utensils, and surgical instruments or dressings.

Vector-borne transmission is when the infection is transmitted from one organism to another. Insects are vectors that transmit disease. An example is mosquitos that transmit West Nile virus.

Infectious diseases can be transmitted through the air in the form of dust and droplets. Dust may contain infectious disease particles in household surfaces and soil. Droplets are tiny particles of infectious disease materials that are formed when sneeze and cough droplets evaporate and float in the air.

Cause and Effect

As epidemiology developed into the scientific discipline that it is today, many people asked what caused diseases. Hippocrates presented a naturalistic approach to disease causation that contradicted religious beliefs of his time. He developed an explanation of cause and effect that focused on changes in the body that were influenced by the environment and heredity.[24] Later in epidemiology's development, Robert Koch suggested that some microscopic agents were the reason people developed disease. Koch presented postulates that resulted in a scientific method to identify those microorganisms that cause disease. Koch's work allowed scientists to identify, isolate, and understand how these microorganisms were related to diseases.

In the twentieth century, the impact of infectious diseases began to decrease as genetic, also referred to as congenital, and chronic diseases became more frequent in the population. This resulted in the need to develop other theories of disease causation. The expansion of the interest and cause and effect of diseases resulted in the use of the concept known as risk. Risk is the probability or how likely it is that someone will get a disease if certain conditions or situations exist. This probability or chance can increase or decrease according to the influence of the conditions or situations that exist. The influencing conditions may be genetic, environmental, behavioral, or a combination of all three.[25]

The link between a cause of disease (a risk factor) and the effect of this cause (the disease) can be thought of in this manner. Before a risk factor can be recognized as a cause of disease, it must be proved that the factor was in the population before a disease occurred. The stronger the association between a risk factor and a disease, the better is the proof that the factor had a role in causing the disease. Methods to measure the strength of an association between a risk factor and a disease will be presented in Chapter Seven. The amount of the risk factor (for example, the number of cigarettes smoked every day) can be used to understand its influence on the development of a disease. If a factor is associated with causing a disease and if it is removed from the population, the risk of disease should decrease. If the association of the risk factor and the disease makes sense biologically, then this adds to the proof that it is a causal factor.

Risk

Risk is a notion that tries to link the effect of factors that may cause a disease. How do we determine if a factor will influence whether someone gets a disease, and if it does, to what extent is this influence weak or strong? Is the factor a strong or weak influence? Does the factor influence the chance of not getting a disease? These are important questions that may not be easy to answer. In fact, we can never be totally sure if a factor does have an influence on the chance of getting a disease. Because of this, epidemiology can only say that there is an association between a disease and its risk factors. Because risk is based on the association between the presence of disease and a risk factor, any or all of the following may be seen: (1) a person who is affected by a risk factor gets the disease, (2) a person who is affected by a risk factor does not get a disease, (3) a person who is not affected by a risk factor gets a disease, and (4) a person who is not affected by a risk factor does not get a disease.

In a population with people who are affected by the same risk factor, the following can happen:

- People who are affected by a risk factor will get the disease. This is when smokers get lung cancer.

- People who are affected by a risk factor will not get the disease. This is when smokers do not get lung cancer.

- People who are not affected by a risk factor will get the disease. This is when people who do not smoke get lung cancer.

- People who are not affected by a risk factor do not get a disease. This is when people who do not smoke do not get lung cancer.

The link between a risk factor and a disease is complex and has been studied for some time. One person who has looked at this link is Rothman.[26] He said that a cause is defined as an act or event that initiates or allows for, by itself or with other factors, a sequence of events that result in an effect, which is the disease. He also said that causes can be classified as either a sufficient or component cause. A *sufficient cause* always produces the disease but is rarely seen in populations. A *component cause*, also called a contributing cause, is one of a group of causes that, when they act together, can be a sufficient cause. The relationship of this group of causes is such that if any one cause is missing, then the person will not get the disease. Most causes of disease are component causes.

Sickle cell disease is an inherited blood disorder that affects an estimated 70,000 to 100,000 Americans. Sickle cell disease is a genetic condition that is present at birth.

Healthy red blood cells are round, and they carry oxygen to all parts of the body. In sickle cell disease, the red blood cells have a different C shape that looks like the farm tool called a sickle.

The sickle cells die early, which causes a constant shortage of red blood cells.

People with sickle cell disease, especially infants and children, are more at risk for harmful infections. Pneumonia is a leading cause of death in infants and young children with sickle cell disease.

Source: Centers for Disease Control and Prevention, http://www.cdc.gov/ncbddd/sicklecell.

The relationship between causes and diseases may be either direct or indirect. *Direct relationship*s are ones in which one factor is directly associated with a disease. This is seen in sickle cell disease, a disease in which infected people have hemoglobin S. In *indirect relationships*, many factors work together in different ways. For example, acute myocardial infarction is known to be caused by high cholesterol levels, thickening of the coronary arteries, and lifestyle behaviors.

Rothman also stated that there are four types of causal relationships. The first type is a necessary and sufficient relationship. In this type, when the factor does not have any influence, a person will not get the disease. In this situation, if the causal factor is absent, the disease will not occur. A classic example is HIV and AIDS. The second type of relationship is necessary but not sufficient. This type has several factors, one of which is required for the disease to occur. An example is tuberculosis in which the bacteria must be present, but exposure to the bacteria is not sufficient to cause the disease. Exposure to *Mycobacterium tuberculosis* will not necessarily result in someone getting tuberculosis because the disease also depends on people having weakened immune systems as well as other factors.

The third type of relationship is sufficient but not necessary. There is a factor that causes a disease, and a person may get a disease even if the factor is not present. This is seen in people with lung cancer who have never smoked. The fourth type is neither sufficient nor necessary. This type is the description of complex models of disease etiology. Examples are a high-fat diet and lifestyle behaviors that are related to heart disease, hypertension, diabetes, and some cancers.

Causation can be presented in the form of a matrix. This matrix can be helpful in understanding the complex relationship between factors that can cause a disease and a person actually getting that disease. Again, because of this complex relationship, the best that epidemiology can offer is whether an association exists between the presence of a factor and the presence of a disease. This association will be quantified later in Chapter Seven, which will show how strong an association is between the factor and a disease.

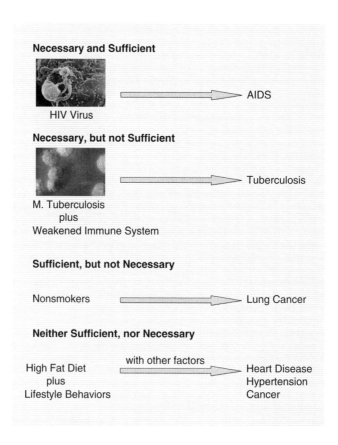

FIGURE 3.2: Causation matrix

	Disease Is Present	Disease Is Absent
Factor Is present	*Situation 1*	*Situation 2*
Factor Is absent	*Situation 3*	*Situation 4*

Figure 3.2 describes in a matrix the four possible relationships between factors and disease. In Situation 1, the disease is present and causal factor is present. In Situation 2, the disease is absent and causal factor is present. In Situation 3, the disease is present (dependent variable) and causal factor is absent (independent variable). In Situation 4, the disease is absent (dependent variable) and causal factor is absent (independent variable).

Web of Causation

Epidemiology has developed a method to describe the relationship between cause and effect by the web of causation.[27] This *web of causation* describes the interconnection of factors that cause a disease. The web works especially well with complex diseases that have many factors that work together to cause a disease. Tuberculosis is a good example in which the web of causation is used to describe the complex relationship between factors and the disease. Tuberculosis factors include exposure to the bacterium that can cause the disease, poor nutrition, living or working in a crowded area, low immunity, and poverty.

Tuberculosis (TB) is a disease caused by the bacterium *Mycobacterium tuberculosis*, which attacks the lungs. The TB bacteria can also attack other parts of the body, including the kidneys, spine, and brain. If not treated properly, TB can result in death.

TB is spread through the air from one person to another, usually through coughing and sneezing.

Latent TB infection occurs when someone is infected but is not sick. The only sign of TB infection is a positive reaction to the tuberculin skin test or special TB blood test. People with latent TB infection are not infectious and cannot spread TB bacteria to others.

Source: Centers for Disease Control and Prevention, http://www.cdc.gov/tb.

FIGURE 3.3: Web of causation

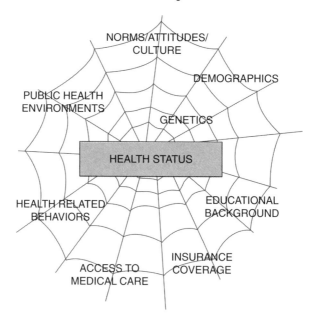

A Web of Factors Contributing to Health Status

The complex nature of the relationship between factors and disease is due to several factors. Factors may need to be present either alone or with other factors. Some factors may be necessary for the disease, and the disease will not occur in the absence of these factors. Several factors working together may be sufficient for disease, but no one factor can cause the disease. The web of causation is the best model to show the relationship to the multiple and interacting causes of chronic diseases. Figure 3.3 shows the web of causation for coronary artery disease.

Because infectious disease study is the basis for all epidemiological principles, epidemiology looks at the relationships between host and environment. A host is a person or vector (insect or animal) in which the infectious agent lives and grows. The host may or may not become sick. A model of this relationship is called the *epidemiological triangle*. Figure 3.4 shows the triangle model. The triangle depicts all aspects of causation, host, environment, and causal agent. Disease development depends on the host's exposure to the agent (or risk factor), the strength of the agent, and the host's susceptibility. Disease development

FIGURE 3.4: Epidemiologic triangle

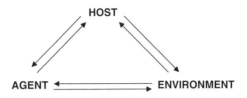

FIGURE 3.5: Wheel of causation

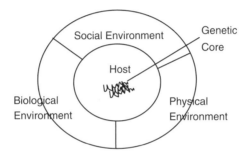

also depends on environmental conditions: biological, social, political, and physical.

Another model that depicts causation is called the wheel. The *wheel of causation model* has a characteristic hub, which is the host. The aspects of the model that surround the hub show the biological, social, and physical determinants of disease. This model has the ability to represent the multiple causes that are common with many diseases. Figure 3.5 shows a wheel of causation.

Summary

In this chapter we discussed health and disease, how they are defined, and their distinction. The natural history of disease was presented with AIDS and diabetes. Disease transmission of infectious diseases was introduced. Disease causation, including the difference between sufficient and necessary causes, was discussed. The web of causation, using coronary artery disease, and the wheel of causation was described. The relationship between causal factors and disease was presented by describing the causation matrix.

Key Terms

Clinical course of a disease, 39

Component cause, 45

Descriptive epidemiology, 39

Direct relationships, 45

Disease, 37

Epidemiological triangle, 48

Health, 36

Health-related quality of life, 38

Hyperglycemia, 39

Indirect relationships, 45

Insulin, 40

Mental health, 36

Natural history of disease, 39

Physical health, 36

Prognosis, 39

Quality of life, 38

Sufficient cause, 45

Underdeveloped country, 40

Vector-borne transmission, 43

Vehicle-borne transmission, 42

Web of causation, 47

Wheel of causation model, 49

Chapter Exercises

1. Define health and disease.
2. Discuss the difference between health and disease.
3. What are the two methods of disease transmission? List the types of indirect transmission.

Chapter Review

1. A person can have a disease but still be considered healthy according to the definition of health. True or False?
2. Determinants of health include
   a. lifestyle.
   b. biological makeup.
   c. environmental conditions.
   d. all of the above.
   e. none of the above.

3. Quality of life measures
   a. body mass index.
   b. overall feeling of well-being.
   c. blood pressure.
   d. none of the above.
4. Understanding the natural history of a disease is helpful in determining
   a. the chance for recovery from a disease.
   b. the future symptoms and outcomes of a disease.
   c. all of the above.
   d. none of the above.
5. Indirect ways that diseases are transmitted include kissing. True or False?
6. Sexually transmitted diseases are spread by direct transmission. True or False?
7. The suggestion that microscopic organisms caused disease was first made by
   a. Hippocrates.
   b. Lind.
   c. Koch.
   d. Graunt.
8. The components of the epidemiological triangle are
   a. host.
   b. environment.
   c. agent.
   d. all of the above.
   e. none of the above.
9. A sufficient cause of a disease always produces the disease. True or False?
10. A component cause of a disease always produces a disease. True or False?

DESCRIBING HEALTH
AND DISEASE

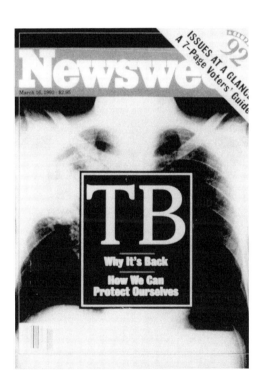

LEARNING OBJECTIVES

On completing this chapter, you will be able to

Describe descriptive epidemiology and its uses
Define a hypothesis and its relationship to descriptive epidemiology
Describe person variables
Describe place variables
Describe time variables
Explain what is meant by an outbreak
Provide examples of uses of descriptive information

Descriptive Epidemiology

Epidemiology as a science is divided into two parts: descriptive and analytical epidemiology. Descriptive epidemiology is involved with identifying and reporting health and disease trends in a population. Descriptive epidemiology tells us to whom, when, and where disease is occurring. Analytical epidemiology, on the other hand, is involved in understanding how and why a disease is occurring. Descriptive and analytical epidemiology work together, with descriptive epidemiology suggesting how and why and analytical epidemiology determining how and why a disease is occurring. *Descriptive epidemiology* is defined as the study of the amount and distribution of disease within a population according to personal variables (age, sex, race, ethnic group, and so on), place variables (country of residence, city of residence, urban area, rural area, areas within a city), and time variables (long-term or short-term trends in health and disease).

Descriptive epidemiology evaluates the impact of disease by identifying trends in a population. These trends may indicate a particular cause of a disease that will then need further study using analytical epidemiology. Descriptive epidemiology is most interested in the frequency and pattern of disease. Knowing the frequency is helpful in evaluating the rate of new cases of a disease. Specific disease patterns tell us about possible causal factors.

Descriptive epidemiology has three general objectives. The first objective is to monitor known diseases and to identify developing disease problems. The second objective is to provide the information that is needed to allocate resources properly. The third objective is to identify those problems that should be further studied using analytical methods.

Hypotheses

The third objective of descriptive epidemiology is to use descriptive information and patterns in data that tell us about factors that may be associated with a disease. This information provides clues to why a disease starts and how it affects people. Descriptive data do not tell us anything about causal relationships. But descriptive data do offer important information regarding health, disease, and disease patterns, illuminating disease patterns in terms of person, place, and time. Descriptive data can help to identify both high-risk groups of individuals for future interventions and problems that should be studied further by analytical epidemiological methods.

The greatest contribution of descriptive epidemiology is that it allows for the development of hypotheses as to why a disease occurs. Descriptive data are valuable because disease does not happen randomly. Instead, it occurs in specific individuals and groups of people in particular geographical areas and during definite periods of time. Describing health and disease in terms of person, place, and time is the foundation for the development of hypotheses. These hypotheses are evaluated by analytical methods that allow for the establishment of the relationship between disease causal factor and disease.

Definition

Descriptive epidemiology is important to developing hypotheses. A *hypothesis* is an educated guess about the relationship between a factor and a disease. After stating a hypothesis, it can be tested to see whether it is true by using some scientific method.

A better definition of a hypothesis is that it is a statement about one or more populations.[1] There are two types of hypotheses: research and statistical. Descriptive epidemiology actually leads to research hypotheses because they are based on observations and opinion that result from experience. A statistical hypothesis, which comes from the more broadly defined research hypotheses, is evaluated using statistical methods. Statistical hypotheses are used in analytical studies, which will be discussed in detail in Chapter Six.

Formulating and Testing Hypotheses

Statistical hypotheses are tested using a scientific method. When developing statistical hypotheses for later testing, two different hypotheses are identified. The first is known as the *null hypothesis*, which is the one that will be tested. The null hypothesis (designated as H_0) states that there is no difference between populations. The other hypothesis is called the *alternative hypothesis* and is designated H_A. The alternative hypothesis contradicts the null hypothesis by stating that the populations are different.

An example of a null hypothesis is the following: the prevalence of diabetes in population A is the same as the prevalence of diabetes in population B. The alternative hypothesis is that the prevalence of diabetes in population A is not the same as in population B. Often a null hypothesis may be stated as follows: the prevalence of diabetes in population A is 12 percent or more. The alternative hypothesis is that the prevalence of diabetes in population A is less than 12 percent. It is important to remember that the null and alternative hypotheses are complements of each other.

To test the null hypothesis (alternative hypotheses are not tested) means that you are attempting to determine if the data support what is stated. The null hypothesis is not tested to see whether or not it is true, but to see whether the information you have can prove what you have stated. Null hypotheses are either accepted (the data support the null hypothesis) or rejected (the data do not support the null hypothesis).

Descriptive Variables

Descriptive variables help to explain which factors affect health and disease. These factors are measured as variables and represent either personal characteristics, where disease is observed (called place), and when and for how long a disease is present (called time). Person factors include age, race, sex, education, and socioeconomic status. Place factors include country, region of a country, county, city, and neighborhoods in a city. Time factors include the season of the year and whether the disease is seen during a short period of time or for many years.

Person

Person characteristics are important in describing health and disease. *Person characteristics* tell us whether a risk factor or a disease is seen more often in one population than in others. Some person characteristics have such a strong association with a disease that they are referred to as *demographic risk factors*. An example is low birth weight's association with the following maternal characteristics: age, race, low socioeconomic status, unmarried, and low level of education.

TABLE 4.1: Limitation of Activity (Percentage) Caused by Chronic Conditions, United States, 2005 and 2006

Age Category, Years	2005	2006
All ages	11.7	11.6
<18	7.0	7.3
18 to 44	5.7	5.5
45 to 54	11.9	12.5
55 to 64	19.9	20.0
≥65	33.8	32.6

Source: Centers for Disease Control and Prevention, *National Vital Statistics Report,* 56(10), April 24, 2008.

The most important person characteristic is age. This is because many diseases are directly related to age, and in general, disease rates are highest in very young and very old people. Disease rates change at different ages. Because of this influence of age, disease rates are often reported as age-specific rates.

Table 4.1 shows the percentage of people who had a limitation of activity as a result of chronic disease in the United States in 2005 and 2006. Overall, there is little difference in the percentage of people who experience a limitation of activity caused by chronic diseases from 2005 through 2006. It is obvious that age is related to limitation of activity. People between the ages of eighteen and forty-four years are less affected by chronic conditions (5.5 percent). The proportion of people who experience a limitation of activity more than doubles at ages forty-five to fifty-four. As people reach the age of fifty-five, the proportion doubles again to 20 percent. At age sixty-five years and older, the percentage increases to a third of the population.

An example of how age affects death is presented in Table 4.2. The death rate from all causes was 847.5 deaths per 100,000 people in the population in 2002. This rate decreased to 825.9 deaths per 100,000 people in the population in 2005. It is easy to see that as age increases, the death rates also increase. The death rate for age categories "<1 year" and "1 to 4 years" is high due to infant mortality and childhood diseases.

In addition to deaths from all causes, age also has an effect on deaths from specific causes. Table 4.3 presents death rates from 2002 to 2005 by age that resulted from diabetes mellitus. From 2002 to 2005 there was little change in the death rate. As was seen in Table 4.3, as people age, the death rate from diabetes mellitus increases. This pattern is seen in almost all diseases.

Age is related to risk factors for many diseases. As people get older, their exposure to risk factors will change. Table 4.4 shows the proportion of people

TABLE 4.2: Death Rates from All Causes by Age,
United States, 2002 to 2005*

Death Rates	2002	2003	2004	2005
All ages, years	847.5	841.9	816.9	825.9
<1	695.0	700.0	685.2	692.5
1 to 4	31.2	31.5	29.9	29.4
5 to 14	17.4	17.0	16.8	16.3
15 to 24	81.4	81.5	80.1	81.4
25 to 34	103.6	103.6	102.1	104.4
35 to 44	202.9	201.6	193.5	193.3
45 to 54	430.1	433.2	427.0	432.0
55 to 64	952.4	940.9	910.3	906.9
65 to 74	2,314.7	2,255.0	2,164.6	2,137.1
75 to 84	5,566.9	5,463.1	5,275.1	5,260.0
≥85	14,828.3	14,593.3	13,823.5	13,798.6

*Per 100,000 population.
Source: Centers for Disease Control and Prevention, *National Vital Statistics Report,*
56(10), April 24, 2008.

TABLE 4.3: Death Rates Caused by Diabetes Mellitus,
by Age, United States, 2002 to 2005*

Death Rates	2002	2003	2004	2005
All ages, years	25.3	25.5	24.9	25.3
<1	—	—	—	—
1 to 4	—	—	—	—
5 to 14	0.1	0.1	0.1	0.1
15 to 24	0.4	0.4	0.4	0.5
25 to 34	1.6	1.6	1.5	1.5
35 to 44	4.8	4.6	4.6	4.7
45 to 54	13.7	13.9	13.4	13.4
55 to 64	37.7	38.5	37.1	37.2
65 to 74	91.4	90.8	87.2	86.8
75 to 84	182.8	181.1	176.9	177.2
≥85	320.6	317.5	307.0	312.1

*Per 100,000 population.
Source: Centers for Disease Control and Prevention, *National Vital Statistics Report,*
56(10), April 24, 2008.

TABLE 4.4: Current Cigarette Smoking Among Adults,
Estimated Percentage, by Sex, United States, 2006

	Total	Men	Women
Age group, year			
19 to 24	28.5	19.3	23.9
25 to 44	26.0	21.0	23.5
45 to 64	24.5	19.3	21.8
≥65	12.6	8.3	10.2

Source: Centers for Disease Control and Prevention. Cigarette smoking among adults, United States, 2006. *Morbidity and Mortality Weekly Report,* November 9, 2007; 56(44): 1157–1161.

TABLE 4.5: Rate of Vision and Hearing Problems
Among People Older Than 18 Years, United States,
Selected Years from 1997 to 2006, by Sex*

Year	Men	Women
1997	88	111
2000	79	101
2004	76	100
2005	79	105
2006	84	105

*Per 1,000 population.
Source: Centers for Disease Control and Prevention, *National Vital Statistics Report,* 56(10), April 24, 2008.

who smoke cigarettes in different age categories. As people get older, the percentage of those who smoke decreases. The percentage of people who smoke decreases from 28.5 percent in the nineteen to twenty-four years age category to 12.6 percent in the sixty-five years and older age category. More women smoke than men in all age categories.

Like age, sex (or gender) has an influence on both disease and death rates in a community. In fact, death rates are higher in men independent of age groups. Disease rates are higher in women, as are the number of comorbidities (having more than one disease at the same time). Because of these differences, disease and death rates are reported as sex-specific rates (for example, male cancer death rate). Table 4.5 presents the sex-specific rate of vision and hearing problems among people older than eighteen years from 1997 to 2006. A

TABLE 4.6: Percentage of Medicaid Coverage
Among People Younger Than 65 Years, United States,
Selected Years from 1984 to 2006, by Sex

	Men	Women
Year		
1984	5.4	8.1
1989	5.7	8.6
1995	9.6	13.4
1997	8.4	11.1
2000	8.2	10.8
2003	10.9	13.6
2004	10.8	13.7
2005	11.6	14.3
2006	12.6	15.5

Source: Centers for Disease Control and Prevention *National Vital Statistics Report,* 56(10), April 24, 2008.

TABLE 4.7: Rate of Hospital Stays in the Past Year,
United States, Selected Years from 1997 to 2006, by Sex*

Year	1997	2005	2006
Men	45	43	42
Women	111	103	96

*Per 1,000 population.
Source: Centers for Disease Control and Prevention, *National Vital Statistics Report,* 56(10), April 24, 2008.

difference can be seen between men and women. Women have a higher rate of vision and hearing problems, which affects their health.

Table 4.6 presents information on Medicaid coverage for people younger than sixty-five (these people are usually not eligible for Medicare, but are considered medically indigent) for selected years from 1984 to 2006. Again, the percentage of women with Medicaid coverage is higher than that of men from 1984 to 2006. Table 4.7 shows the rate of hospitalization in the United States from 1997 and 2006. As expected, the rate of hospitalization for women is more than two times higher than for men.

WHAT DOES MEDICALLY INDIGENT MEAN?

A person is considered to be **medically indigent** if he or she does not have private health insurance and is not eligible for governmental health insurance, including Medicare and Medicaid. People who are medically indigent usually work, but they do not have private insurance, earn too much money to qualify for Medicaid, and are too young to be eligible for Medicare.

Source: Weitz R. *The sociology of health, illness and health care: A critical approach,* 4th ed. Thomson/Wadsworth, 2009.

As with age and sex, disease patterns are affected by race and ethnic group membership. Race affects both how often disease occurs (the frequency of disease) and how severely (the magnitude of the effect) disease affects people in a population. Research tells us that African Americans have much higher death rates from hypertensive heart disease, cerebrovascular accidents, tuberculosis, syphilis, homicide, and accidental death than other racial and ethnic groups. On the other hand, whites have much higher death rates from arteriosclerotic heart disease, suicide, and leukemia. These differences indicate that disease and death are influenced by race.

The death rate for all causes is higher in whites and is significantly higher for diseases of the heart, suicide, malignant neoplasms, and Alzheimer's disease. Table 4.8 shows age-adjusted death rates by race in the United States from 2002

TABLE 4.8: Age-Adjusted Death Rates by Race, United States, 2002 to 2005*

	All Races	White	Black	American Indian or Alaska Native	Asian or Pacific Islander
Year					
2002	847.3	895.7	768.4	403.6	299.5
2003	841.9	890.1	763.6	422.6	303.9
2004	816.5	863.2	744.3	416.8	297.2
2005	825.9	873.7	749.4	440.3	307.7

*Per 100,000 population.
Source: Centers for Disease Control and Prevention, *National Vital Statistics Report,* 56(10), April 24, 2008.

TABLE 4.9: Rate of Emergency Room Visits in the
Past Year for Persons Younger Than 18 Years,
United States, Selected Years from 1997 to 2006, by Race*

Year	1997	2005	2006
White	194	198	212
Black	240	238	250
Asian	126	146	134
American Indian or Alaska Native	241	321	197
Hispanic	211	195	197

*Per 1,000 population.
Source: Centers for Disease Control and Prevention, *National Vital Statistics Report,* 56(10), April 24, 2008.

to 2005. The age-adjusted death rate for all races has decreased from 847.3 deaths per 100,000 people in the population in 2002 to 825.9 deaths per 100,000 people in the population. When each race is reviewed and compared with other races, a clear difference is seen. First, the age-adjusted death rate has not changed significantly in each racial group from 2002 to 2005. In 2002 whites had the highest age-adjusted death rate of 895.7 deaths per 100,000 people in the population, much higher than blacks (768.4), American Indians or Alaska Natives (403.6), and Asians or Pacific Islanders (299.5). This pattern in age-adjusted death rates continued from 2002 until 2005. In 2005 whites had the highest age-adjusted death rate (873.7 per 100,000 people in the population), followed by blacks (749.4), American Indians or Alaska Natives (440.3), and Asians or Pacific Islanders (307.7).

Table 4.9 presents the rate of emergency room visits for children younger than eighteen years during 1997 to 2006. This information highlights the differences in the rate of emergency room visits for each racial group. In 1997 blacks (240 visits per 1,000 people in the population) and American Indians or Alaska Natives (241 visits per 1,000 people in the population) had the highest rate of emergency room visits. Asians had the lowest rate of 126 visits per 1,000 people in the population. In 2006 the rate for blacks was still the highest (250 visits per 1,000 people in the population), but whites now had the second highest rate (212 visits per 1,000 people in the population). Again, Asians had the lowest rate of 134 visits per 1,000 people in the population.

Table 4.10 presents the percentage of teenaged childbearing in the United States from 2002 to 2005. In all races, the percentage has remained basically the same. Black teenagers had more pregnancies in all years, except for 2005.

TABLE 4.10: Percentage of Teenaged Childbearing,
United States, 2002 to 2006, by Race

Year	All Races	White	Black	American Indian or Alaska Native	Asian	Hispanic
2002	3.3	3.1	6.9	3.6	1.1	5.6
2003	3.4	3.0	6.6	6.6	1.1	5.4
2004	3.4	3.0	6.4	6.4	1.1	5.4
2005	3.4	2.9	6.2	6.5	1.0	5.3

Source: Centers for Disease Control and Prevention, *National Vital Statistics Report,* 56(10), April 24, 2008.

TABLE 4.11: Percentage of People Older Than 18 Years
with Vision and Hearing Problems, United States,
Selected Years from 1997 to 2006, by Race

Year	White	Black	American Indian/Alaska Native	Asian	Hispanic
1997	9.7	12.8	19.2	6.2	10.0
2000	8.8	10.6	16.6	6.3	9.7
2004	8.8	10.3	14.8	5.1	8.8
2005	9.1	10.9	14.9	5.5	9.6
2006	9.5	10.4	16.7	7.0	9.9

Source: Centers for Disease Control and Prevention, *National Vital Statistics Report,* 56(10), April 24, 2008.

The percentage in blacks steadily decreased. Asians had the lowest percentage of teenaged pregnancies, with whites having the second lowest during the four-year period.

To further show how race affects disease, Table 4.11 presents the percentage of people with vision and hearing problems in adults. The highest percentage is seen in American Indians or Alaska Natives. Asians had the lowest percentage, with whites and Hispanics having similar percentages. It is interesting to see how much higher the percentage is among American Indians or Alaska Natives. This difference indicates that there must be something in either the biological or cultural makeup of American Indians or Alaska Natives that causes this difference.

Socioeconomic status is a term that is often referred to as social class but is related to several different personal characteristics, including occupation, income, education, and total lifestyle. In fact, in public health the preferred term for social class is socioeconomic status. Socioeconomic status is directly related to health and disease, and the following is typically seen: as the socioeconomic status declines, disease and death rates increase.

It is known that the level of educational attainment (the number of completed years of formal education) has an influence on survival from cancers. The less educated someone is, the poorer that person's chances for cancer survival. In addition, research on the relationship between educational attainment and death rates has revealed some interesting information. Death rates are higher in groups with lower educational attainment. For example, as socioeconomic status and educational level increase, coronary heart disease mortality rates decrease.

The incidence in many diseases has been related to socioeconomic status. An example is the risk of end-stage renal disease, which is significantly higher in blacks than in whites. This difference between races is less, but still exists, after adjusting for socioeconomic status.[2]

Table 4.12 shows the age-adjusted death rates for people between the ages of twenty-five and sixty-four, using educational attainment as a measure of socioeconomic status. People with less than high school education have the highest age-adjusted death rate, meaning they died more frequently than people with more than a high school education. Their death rate has increased from

TABLE 4.12: Age-Adjusted Death Rates Among Persons Aged 25 to 64 Years by Educational Attainment, Selected States, 2001 to 2005*

Year	2001	2002	2003	2004	2005
Education					
Less than high school	576.6	575.1	669.9	667.2	650.4
High school graduate	480.9	490.9	490.9	477.1	477.6
Some college or higher	214.6	211.3	211.7	208.3	206.3

*Per 100,000 population.
Source: Centers for Disease Control and Prevention, *National Vital Statistics Report,* 56(10), April 24, 2008.

TABLE 4.13: Percentage of People Older Than 18 Years
with Vision and Hearing Problems, United States,
Selected Years from 1997 to 2006, by Educational Attainment

	No High School or GED	High School Diploma or GED	Some College or More
Year			
1997	15.0	10.6	8.9
2000	12.2	9.5	8.9
2004	13.8	10.3	7.9
2005	13.5	10.3	9.2
2006	12.9	10.6	9.2

Source: Centers for Disease Control and Prevention, *National Vital Statistics Report,* 56(10), April 24, 2008.

2001 (576.6 deaths per 100,000 people in the population) to 2005 (650.4 deaths per 100,000 people in the population). The lowest death rate is seen in people with some college or higher. Their death rate has decreased from 2001 (214.6 deaths per 100,000 people in the population) to 2005 (206.3 deaths per 100,000 people in the population).

Table 4.13 shows the effect of the level of educational attainment on disease. People who are not high school graduates nor have a general equivalency diploma had the highest percentage of adults with vision and hearing problems. This group's percentage has decreased from 1997 to 2006, but it still remained the highest. People with some college or more had the lowest percentage with vision and hearing problems.

Place

Place is another important descriptor of health and disease. Place indicates several specific characteristics of a geographical area. These characteristics are used to compare countries, regions of the world, urban and rural areas, and areas within a city. The characteristics that are represented by place indicate work conditions, number of people in a community (known as population density), and environmental conditions. Place is used to understand whether a disease is clustered in one geographical area, which indicates specific place conditions. Different areas, identified by natural boundaries, usually have differing frequencies of specific diseases. This results from specific environmental factors. In fact, diseases whose occurrence depends on specific environmental conditions are called *place diseases*. An example is malaria, which is seen in specific areas in the world.

TABLE 4.14: Estimated TB Incidence Rate for Selected Countries, 2006*

Country	Incidence Rate	Country	Incidence Rate
Afghanistan	161	Iraq	56
Argentina	39	Italy	7
Bangladesh	225	Mexico	21
Belgium	13	New Zealand	9
Bulgaria	40	Peru	162
China	99	Poland	25
Cuba	9	Senegal	270
Egypt	24	Spain	30
Finland	5	Turkey	29
France	14	United States	4
India	168		

*Per 100,000 population.
Source: World Health Organization, 2010, http://www.who.int/topics/tuberculosis/en/.

Different disease rates can be seen across countries. Table 4.14 presents rates for tuberculosis in several countries. You can easily see that the rates are different in the countries listed. Senegal, in Western Africa, has the highest TB incidence rate of 270 cases per 100,000 people in the population. Bangladesh has the second highest incidence rate of 225 cases per 100,000 people in the population. Both Senegal and Bangladesh are poor, developing countries. Developed, richer countries have a much lower incidence rate for TB. The United States has the lowest incidence rate (4 cases per 100,000 people in the population), closely followed by Finland and Italy. Again, the unique characteristics of these countries account for the low incidence rates.

A region of a country may have different rates of disease than other regions. Table 4.15 shows average annual age-adjusted death rates from 2003 to 2005 in different regions in the United States. The overall average annual age-adjusted death rate in the United States was 892.0 deaths per 100,000 people in the population. When the United States is divided into nine regions, very different death rates are seen. The Pacific region has the lowest rate, 733.0 deaths per 100,000 people in the population. The East South Central region has the highest rate of 985.6 deaths per 100,000 people in the population. All the regions except the East South Central and the West South Central have lower rates than the total rate for the entire country. Because these rates have been standardized to eliminate the effect of difference in ages in the different regions, Table 4.15

TABLE 4.15: Average Annual Age-Adjusted Death Rates, Regions of the United States, 2003 to 2005*

Region	2003–2005
United States	892.0
New England	742.7
Middle Atlantic	771.4
East North Central	828.1
West North Central	784.4
South Atlantic	834.2
East South Central	985.6
West South Central	892.0
Mountain	788.5
Pacific	733.0

*Per 100,000 population.
Source: Centers for Disease Control and Prevention, National Center for Health Statistics, National Vital Statistics System, 2005.

TABLE 4.16: Average Annual Age-Adjusted Death Rates by Selected States, 2003 to 2005*

State	2003–2005
Arizona	775.2
California	727.2
Florida	765.9
Georgia	943.7
Hawaii	623.6
Iowa	748.0
Maine	816.7
Massachusetts	745.6
Mississippi	1,022.4
New Jersey	762.7
Ohio	862.5
South Carolina	960.4
Texas	846.2

*Per 100,000 population.
Source: Centers for Disease Control and Prevention, National Center for Health Statistics, National Vital Statistics System, 2005.

indicates that there are other explanations for the variability in rates. These explanations include differences in poverty rates, lifestyle behaviors, and other factors that are related to death.

As might be expected, these differences are also seen among states, counties, cities, and within cities. Table 4.16 shows average annual age-adjusted death rates from 2003 to 2005 in selected states in the United States. Hawaii had the

TABLE 4.17: County-Level Estimated Diagnosed Diabetes,
by Selected Counties in Mississippi, 2005

County	Percentage
Coahoma	14.0
De Soto	13.4
Holmes	14.5
Jackson	11.0
Kemper	13.7
Lamar	8.4
Lee	10.9
Quitman	13.4
Rankin	8.3
Union	9.8

Source: Mississippi State Department of Health, Division of Statistics, 2005.

lowest death rate of 623.6 deaths per 100,000 people in the population. Mississippi had the highest rate (1,022.4 deaths per 100,000 people in the population). As was seen in Table 4.15 above, states in the Western part of the United States, California and Arizona, had lower rates. States in the Southern and Southeastern parts of the United States (Mississippi, Georgia, South Carolina, and Texas) had higher rates. Explanations for this difference are the same as they were above: differences in poverty rates, lifestyle behaviors, and other factors that are related to death.

Let's take a closer look at Mississippi, which had the highest age-adjusted death rates in Table 4.16. Table 4.17 presents estimated percentages for diagnosed diabetes, one of the fifteen leading causes of death in selected counties in Mississippi in 2006. The table shows that there are very different diabetes percentages across the state. Rankin County, which is near the state capital, had the lowest percentage of people with diabetes. Lamar County, which is in the south central part of the state, had the second lowest percentage of people with diabetes. Holmes County, in the Mississippi Delta region, had the highest percentage. De Soto County, which is near Memphis, had a high percentage of people with diabetes. This comparison tells us that even in the same state, death and disease rates may differ because of *place characteristics*.

Urban and rural areas have different disease rates. Table 4.18 lists rates for age-adjusted death rates for urban and rural areas from 1996 to 2005. In the United States, rates have decreased since 1996, but the rates remain higher in rural areas. If we look at the regions of the United States, the highest death rates in urban areas is in the Midwest. The highest death rates in rural areas are seen

TABLE 4.18: Average Annual Age-Adjusted Death Rates,
Urban and Rural Counties, United States, 1996–1998,
1999–2001, and 2003–2005*

	1996–1998	1999–2001	2003–2005
United States			
Urban	894.5	869.0	794.2
Rural	913.0	907.1	886.4
Northeast			
Urban	909.6	861.7	779.9
Rural	878.4	854.4	812.7
Midwest			
Urban	951.7	939.6	863.6
Rural	868.6	865.2	819.1
South			
Urban	938.1	926.8	847.7
Rural	974.1	973.3	935.1
West			
Urban	819.2	792.4	727.8
Rural	861.0	851.8	815.3

*Per 100,000 population.
Source: Centers for Disease Control and Prevention, *National Vital Statistics Report,*
56(10), April 24, 2008.

in the South. This table shows that death rates are very different and have been higher in rural areas from 1996 to 2005.

Time

Time patterns can show when disease happens and help us to understand the characteristics of the disease progression. Patterns include short term and long term. Disease happens in cycles, seasonally, in epidemics, and in long-term secular trends. Time helps to understand specific diseases and indicates whether people will need medical services. The incidence and prevalence of flu and pneumonia are higher in the months of November through February, so medical providers can prepare for treating affected people. When diseases appear at times that are unexpected, then we are alerted that a problem may be occurring.

An endemic is a period of time when the expected number cases of a disease is seen. An *epidemic* (also called an *outbreak*) is an unexpected increase in the number of cases of a disease at a specific time and place or among a specific subpopulation. For example, historically AIDS was first identified because of the unexpected cases of pneumococcal pneumonia and Kaposi's sarcoma among young men. Epidemics are easily identified by a graph of the number of cases over a period of time. This graph is called an *epidemic curve*. The graph characterizes a short-term trend that shows the number of cases that happen over a few hours, days, weeks, or months.

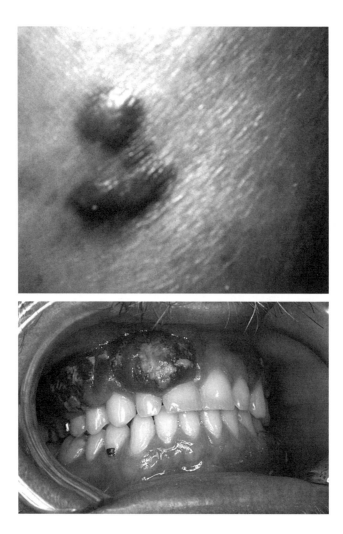

There are two types of epidemics, which are indicated by the shape of the curve. A *point-exposure epidemic*, which is caused by the same exposure at the same point in time and happens over a period of days, will result in a steep, peaked curve. Food poisoning and gastrointestinal problems are examples of point-exposure epidemics. A *propagated epidemic*, which is caused by different exposures over a long period and lasts for years, has a less steep curve. AIDS is an example of a propagated epidemic. Figures 4.1 and 4.2 present a point-exposure and a propagated epidemic.

Disease trends sometimes follow seasons of the year. Some diseases are expected to happen in the winter, and some diseases are expected in summer months. Because these seasonal fluctuations in the number of cases are expected, this is not an epidemic (remember the definition given earlier: an epidemic is an unexpected increase in the incidence of disease). But understanding that diseases will occur in different seasons of the year is helpful for providing necessary health care services for a community.

OVERWEIGHT AND OBESITY

The *body mass index* (BMI) is used to measure overweight and obesity in adults. The BMI is a number calculated using a person's weight and height. The following BMI ranges are for overweight and obesity:

- An adult who has a BMI between 25 and 29.9 is considered overweight.

- An adult who has a BMI of 30 or higher is considered obese.

For children and teens (ages two to nineteen years), BMI ranges are defined so that they take into account normal differences in body fat between boys and girls and differences in body fat at various ages. The BMI value is plotted on the Centers for Disease Control and Prevention (CDC) growth charts to determine the corresponding BMI-for-age percentile.

- Overweight is defined as a BMI at or above the 85th percentile and lower than the 95th percentile.

- Obesity is defined as a BMI at or above the 95th percentile for children of the same age and sex

Source: Centers for Disease Control and Prevention. http://www.cdc.gov/obesity/index.html.

Why do diseases follow seasons of the year? These seasonal diseases are affected by the way they are transmitted between people. For example,

FIGURE 4.1: Point-source epidemic

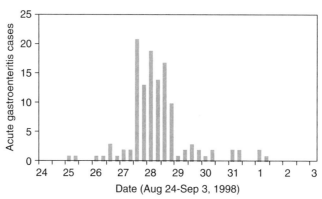

Source: Centers for Disease Control and Prevention.

FIGURE 4.2: Propagated epidemic: Estimated number of AIDS cases in adults and adolescents, United States, 1985 to 2006

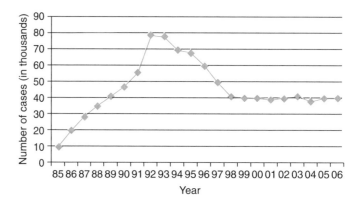

Source: Centers for Disease Control and Prevention.

chickenpox, which affects school-aged children, usually occurs in winter months. Chickenpox is seasonal because schoolchildren remain indoors for long periods each day in the winter, so this communicable infection is easily transmitted in close quarters. Flu is another seasonal disease that happens mostly in winter months. The seasonal nature of flu allows physicians' offices, clinics, and hospitals to stock up on flu vaccine and to predict hospital staffing needs that will result from the admission of highly susceptible individuals. Some dermatological diseases follow seasonal variation. Dyschromia and seborrheic keratosis are seen mostly in the spring and summer months. Acne and folliculitis are most often seen in fall and winter months.[3] Figure 4.3 shows a seasonal disease graph.

Diseases that are presented over a long period of time are monitored in secular trends. These long-term patterns in disease are studied to understand the effects of the disease presence for such a long time. Figure 4.4 shows a secular trend for hospitalizations associated with *Clostridium difficile* infection in Finland. The incidence was monitored from 1996 to 2004. The pattern indicates that the incidence for hospitalization primarily due to *C. difficile* infection K52.8 has significantly increased from 1996 to 2004.[4]

CROHN'S DISEASE

Crohn's disease is a chronic inflammation in the bowel resulting from immune system malfunction. Research indicates that in people with Crohn's disease, the immune system, which is responsible for protecting the body from invading substances, actually mistakes some bacteria and other organisms normally found in the intestines for foreign invaders. The body then sends white blood cells into the lining of the intestines to fight these so-called invaders. This overproduction of white blood cells results in the inflammation of the intestines. Prolonged inflammation can lead to ulcerations and injury to portions of the bowel.

The most common initial symptoms of Crohn's disease are abdominal pain, cramping, and diarrhea. Pain usually arises at or below the navel, often in the lower right portion of the abdomen. These symptoms tend to show up after meals. Other symptoms may include: loss of appetite, rectal bleeding, weight loss, fever, joint pain, fatigue, anal skin tags, and fistulas.

Source: Centocor Ortho Biotech Inc. Web site: https://www.livingwithcrohnsdisease.com/livingwithcrohnsdisease/index.html.

Other Descriptive Variables

The risk of health and disease in a population is important information for scientists and health service managers. The Behavioral Risk Factor Surveillance System (BRFSS) is a large telephone survey, conducted by each state and administered by the CDC, that is used to plan for the provision of health services to

FIGURE 4.3: Seasonal disease graph

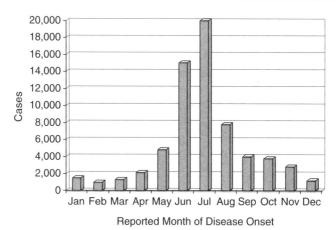

Source: Centers for Disease Control and Prevention, MMWR, Vol. 49, No. SS-3

FIGURE 4.4: Secular trend of hospitalizations associated with *Clostridium difficile* infection in Finland, 1996 to 2004

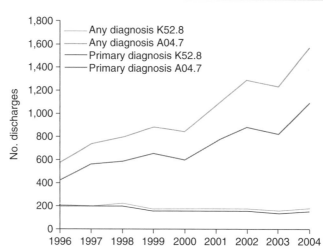

Source: Centers for Disease Control and Prevention. Lyytikäinen O, Turunen H, Sund R, Rasinperä M, Könönen E, Ruutu P, et al. Hospitalizations and deaths related to *Clostridium difficile* infection, Finland, 1996–2004. *Emerg Infect Dis* [serial on the Internet]. 2009 May [*date cited*]. Available from http://www.cdc.gov/EID/content/15/5/761.htm

improve the health of people in the United States. The BRFSS started in 1984 as statewide surveys, with several states stratifying information to understand region-specific data trends within states. The scope of the BRFSS is adults and their personal health behaviors that are thought to affect health and disease. These personal health behaviors are considered to be linked with chronic diseases and include lack of physical activity, overweight, poor nutrition, tobacco and alcohol use, and nonuse of preventive health services.[5]

An extension of the BRFSS is the Youth Risk Behavior Surveillance System (YRBSS). The YRBSS was established in 1990 to survey youths and young adults who are not included in the BRFSS. The YRBSS is focused on health behaviors that affect the causes of death, disability, and social problems among youths and young adults in the United States. Behaviors of interest include tobacco, alcohol, and drug use; dietary behaviors; lack of physical activity; sexual behaviors; and behaviors that may result in unintentional injury or violence. The purpose of the YRBSS includes estimating the prevalence of health-risk behaviors, documenting trends in health-risk distribution over time, and studying the co-occurrence of health behaviors using national and state comparisons and subpopulation comparisons.[6]

Examples of Use of Descriptive Information

Secular trends have been studied for many years to identify the pattern of disease over a period of many years. One example is the study of factors that cause heart disease and their relationship to body weight.[7] According to the study by Gregg and colleagues, the prevalence of obesity has increased but the changes in heart disease risk factors were not known. So the study was done to measure the change in heart disease risk factors in people with different body weights and body mass index (BMI).

The results of the study were that all risk factors, except for diabetes, have decreased at all BMI levels. The largest change was seen in people who are considered overweight and obese. Specifically, 21 percent less people had high cholesterol levels, and 18 percent less had high blood pressure compared with the proportion forty years ago. In addition, 12 percent less people were smokers. Obese people still have more risk factors than others; the levels of these risk factors have decreased over the past forty years.

Another example is the study of the influence of excess body weight on patient outcomes after myocardial infarction. This study evaluated the prevalence of overweight and obese people who had a myocardial infarction. The study found that almost 65 percent of people who had a myocardial infarction were overweight or obese. This percentage has increased since 1978. The study also found that overweight and obese people were more likely to have other risk factors, like high cholesterol levels, high blood pressure, and diabetes. The conclusions of the study included that the prevalence of overweight and obese people among those who had a myocardial infarction was high and that this percentage had increased over the past thirty years.

Summary

In this chapter, we introduced and defined descriptive epidemiology. Descriptive epidemiology tells to whom, when, and where disease is occurring. Descriptive epidemiology suggests reasons why disease is occurring and why it isn't in other populations. Descriptive information allows for formulating hypotheses that can be tested to see the relationship between risk factors and disease.

Descriptive epidemiology variables include person, place, and time characteristics. Age is the person variable that has the largest effect on health and disease. A greater frequency of disease is seen in the very young and very old. Race and sex also have a significant influence on health and disease.

Place diseases were discussed. Malaria is a place disease because it is seen in specific places in the world. Epidemics are unexpected increases in the number of new cases of disease, and they may occur over short or long durations. Some diseases occur at different times of the year, and they are called seasonal diseases.

Key Terms

Alternative hypothesis, 56

Body mass index, 71

Crohn's disease, 73

Descriptive epidemiology, 54

Epidemic, 69

Epidemic curve, 70

Hypothesis, 55

Null hypothesis, 55

Outbreak, 69

Person characteristics, 56

Place characteristics, 68

Place diseases, 65

Point exposure epidemic, 70

Propagated epidemic, 71

Socioeconomic status, 64

Statistical hypotheses, 55

Time patterns, 69

Chapter Exercises

1. Describe the difference between point-exposure epidemics and propagated epidemics. Give an example of each.
2. What is the difference between the conditions overweight and obesity?
3. What is the definition of an outbreak?

Chapter Review

1. Descriptive epidemiology
   a. can be used to identify specific etiological factors that are investigated in analytical studies.
   b. is the study of the distribution of disease by characteristics of person, place, and time.
   c. makes use of readily available information from vital statistics and censuses.
   d. all of the above.
   e. none of the above.

Answer True or False to Questions 2 through 10

2. Descriptive epidemiology evaluates the impact of disease by identifying trends in a population.
3. An epidemic is an unusual increase in the incidence rate of a disease.
4. Death rates are the same across different age groups.
5. Disease rates are different for different racial groups.
6. Socioeconomic factors usually do not affect the occurrence of disease.
7. An increase of pneumonia cases at a hospital in January is indicative of an epidemic.
8. The AIDS epidemic is an example of a propagated epidemic.
9. Information from descriptive studies can be used to test hypotheses about cause-and-effect relationships.
10. The alternative hypothesis states that there is no difference between the study groups.

MEASURING HEALTH
AND DISEASE

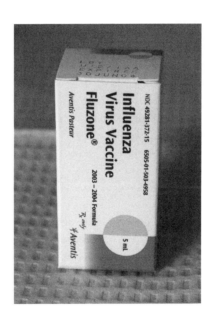

LEARNING OBJECTIVES

On completing this chapter, you will be able to

Explain the use of counts
Discuss what is a rate
Define incidence rate
Define prevalence rate
Discuss the distinction between and uses of incidence and prevalence rates
Discuss the importance of rates
Describe mortality rates
Construct a graph of health and disease information
Discuss the concept of confounding

Morbidity

Morbidity means illness or the state of having a disease. One definition of morbidity is the rate of the development of new cases of a disease. So morbidity allows us to understand how much disease is in a population and how fast it develops. Morbidity is measured using two epidemiological measures: incidence rate and prevalence rate.

A *rate* is defined as the number of people having a disease during a specific time period, divided by the total number of people in the population who could develop this disease. Rates can also measure the number of people with a specific characteristic or trait (for example, smokers) during a period of time, again divided by all the people in a population. Rates are usually multiplied by some factor, typically a multiple of ten, so it is easier to understand any differences between populations. Rates are usually written as a percentage or events per number of people in a population (per 1,000, per 10,000, or per 100,000 people). Several rates have characteristic formats, such as infant and neonatal mortality rates, which are expressed as the rate per 1,000 live births. Birth and death rates are presented per 100,000 people in a population. Age-specific and cause-specific death rates are expressed as the rate per 100,000 people in the population.

The basic form of a *morbidity rate* is

$$\frac{\text{number of cases of a disease or condition in a population during a specified period of time}}{\text{number of people in a population during a specified period of time}}$$

TABLE 5.1: AIDS Rates in the United States in 2006
by Race or Ethnic Group

Race or Ethnic Group	Rate (per 100,000 people)
White, not Hispanic	11.2
Black, not Hispanic	82.9
Hispanic	31.3
Asian or Pacific Islander	7.5
American Indian or Alaska Native	12.2

Source: Centers for Disease Control and Prevention, http://www.cdc.gov/hiv/resources/factsheets/index.htm.

The numerator of a rate consists of the cases that have been identified from routinely collected data or data from specifically designed studies. Denominators of rates are usually the total number of people in a population, which comes from the U.S. Census. Table 5.1 presents the rate of AIDS cases in the United States in 2006, by racial or ethnic group.

Ratios are also used to measure morbidity. A ratio compares the numerator with the denominator. For example, the male-to-female ratio compares males in the numerator with females in the denominator. In ratios the numerator is not included in the denominator. However, in a rate the number in the numerator is always included as part of the number in the denominator. Ratios are expressed as a number to 1 (for example, 5 to 1, which may be written 5:1). If the number of deaths from diabetes in males was 100 and the number of deaths from diabetes in females is 50, then the ratio would be 2 to 1 (or 2:1). As with rates, some unit of time (a particular year, for example) is used with ratios.

Another way to measure disease is to use a count. A *count* is simply the number of people who have a disease or a specific trait. Counts are not used to compare populations, but they can be used to identify how many people in a population have a specific disease during a period of time. Counts are the simplest method of measuring disease frequency. As an example, Table 5.2 presents the absolute number of cumulative cases of AIDS in the United States up to 2006, according to age. Without population numbers (as are seen in rates), comparisons cannot be made about which age category has the greatest rate of AIDS, nor can you make comparisons with other populations. Table 5.3 shows the cumulative reported AIDS deaths through 2006 in the United States.

TABLE 5.2: Cumulative Reported AIDS Cases Through 2006 in the United States

	Number of Cases
Adults and adolescents	983,343
Children younger than 13 years	9,522
Total	992,865

Source: Centers for Disease Control and Prevention, http://www.cdc.gov/hiv/resources/factsheets/index.htm.

TABLE 5.3: Cumulative Reported AIDS Deaths Through 2006 in the United States

	Number of Deaths
Adults and adolescents	544,015
Children younger than 13 years	5,579
Total	549,594

Source: Centers for Disease Control and Prevention, http://www.cdc.gov/hiv/resources/factsheets/index.htm.

Incidence

Incidence (it is not necessary to use the word *rate* with incidence, because incidence is a rate) follows one of the morbidity definitions. *Incidence* is the rate at which new cases of a disease develop in a population. Incidence helps to explain how fast a disease develops. Incidence is a rate, which means that it measures the new cases during a precisely defined time period in a population. Incidence can be thought of as a way of measuring the risk that a person in a population has of getting a disease during a specified time period.

Incidence is a measure that expresses the continual occurrence of new cases of a disease or condition and may be defined as

$$\frac{\text{number of new cases of a disease or condition}}{\text{in a specific population over a specified period of time}}$$
$$\frac{}{\text{total number of people at risk of developing a}}$$
disease in a specific population over a specified period of time

The denominator is usually the average number of people in a population at the midpoint of the period, which is important. For example, an incidence rate for six months should be evaluated differently from an incidence rate for six years. You should expect more new cases in a six-year period than in a six-month period. The specified period of time must be the same in both the numerator and denominator.

To better understand the specified time period used, you should think of incidence as the number of new cases that occur between two points in time, t_0 to t_1. The time period starts at t_0 (for example, today is t_0) and it continues until t_1 (possibly one year from today). All new occurrences of a disease between t_0 (today) and t_1 (one year from today) are measured and are used as the numerator for the incidence rate. The total population at risk between t_0 and t_1 is used as the denominator. The people in the denominator could possibly develop the disease during the specific time period that is used to measure incidence.

To provide an example of calculating incidence rates, consider the following situation that concerns patients discharged from a hospital with complications due to diabetes. Five patients are tracked from the day of discharge (t_0) for a five-year period (the fifth year is t_1) to determine if they will be readmitted to the hospital. During the five-year period, two patients are readmitted and the remaining three patients are not readmitted. The incidence rate is 2 cases per 5 people over a five-year period. This equals an incidence of 40 percent, or forty readmissions per one hundred patients.

An example of the use of incidence is shown in Table 5.4. Table 5.4 presents crude incidence rates of invasive cancers by primary site in the United States in 2004. The incidence rates are categorized (also known as stratified) by race and ethnicity: whites, blacks, and Hispanics. The incidence rate for all cancers in 2004 was 489.5 per 100,000 people in the population. The highest incidence rate was seen in cancers in the male genital system (139.5), and the lowest was Kaposi's sarcoma (0.8). It is interesting to look at the differences in incidence rates in the different racial and ethnic groups. Using male genital system cancers as a comparison, the incidence is equal in whites and blacks.[1]

However, the incidence in whites and blacks is almost three times higher than the rate in Hispanics. This same difference is seen in cancers of the respiratory system and the oral cavity and pharynx. Cancer incidence rates at the primary sites of the skin, urinary system, brain, and endocrine system, and of lymphomas and leukemia, are much higher in whites than blacks and Hispanics. Cancer incidence of myelomas is highest in blacks.

Another example of the use of incidence is shown in Tables 5.5 and 5.6. Table 5.5 presents incidence rates of acute hepatitis A by state from 2002 to 2006. Overall, the incidence has decreased over the five-year period. The incidence of acute hepatitis A over the five-year period was highest in Arizona, with

TABLE 5.4: Crude Invasive Cancer Incidence Rates* by Primary Site and Race and Ethnicity, United States, 2004

Cancer Type	All Races	Whites	Blacks	Hispanics
All Sites	489.5	510.7	389.6	188.3
Oral cavity and pharynx	15.1	15.7	12.8	5.2
Digestive system	95.0	97.7	82.8	45.7
Respiratory system	84.2	88.8	73.1	22.2
Bones and joints	1.0	1.0	0.8	0.8
Soft tissue including heart	3.4	3.5	2.6	2.2
Skin excluding basal and squamous	21.6	24.8	1.3	2.6
Male genital system	139.5	138.9	139.1	54.9
Breast	1.3	1.3	1.2	0.4
Urinary system	51.5	57.1	24.7	16.8
Eye and orbit	0.9	1.0	0.2	0.1
Brain and other nervous system	7.4	8.2	3.7	4.1
Endocrine system	5.3	5.7	2.5	2.8
Lymphomas	23.7	25.4	14.8	12.3
Myeloma	6.1	5.9	8.1	2.8
Leukemias	13.7	14.7	8.0	7.0
Mesothelioma	1.7	1.9	0.6	0.6
Kaposi's sarcoma	0.8	0.7	1.5	1.2
Miscellaneous	17.3	18.4	11.8	6.5

*Per 100,000 population.
Source: U.S. Cancer Statistics Working Group, United States Cancer Statistics: 1999–2004 Incidence and Mortality Web-based Report. Atlanta: U.S. Department of Health and Human Services, Centers for Disease Control and Prevention and National Cancer Institute; 2007.

TABLE 5.5: Incidence of Acute Hepatitis A by Selected States in the United States, 2002 to 2006*

State	2002	2003	2004	2005	2006
Arizona	5.6	5.0	4.6	3.3	2.9
California	4.1	3.2	2.5	2.4	2.7
Delaware	1.9	1.1	0.7	0.7	1.5
Massachusetts	2.2	3.4	10.3	4.5	1.3
New Hampshire	0.9	1.5	2.1	6.3	1.7
Rhode Island	3.2	1.6	2.2	1.8	1.5
Texas	3.9	2.8	2.8	2.0	1.4

*Rate per 100,000 population.
Source: National Notifiable Diseases Surveillance System, 1996 to 2006: http://www.cdc.gov/hepatitis/statistics.htm.

TABLE 5.6: Incidence Rates* of Actual Viral Hepatitis by Type and Year, United States, 1997 to 2006

Year	Hepatitis A	Hepatitis B	Hepatitis C or Non-A, Non-B
1997	11.2	3.9	1.4
1998	8.6	3.8	1.3
1999	6.3	2.8	1.1
2000	4.8	2.9	1.1
2001	3.7	2.8	0.7
2002	3.1	2.8	0.5
2003	2.6	2.6	0.3
2004	1.9	2.1	0.3
2005	1.5	1.8	0.2
2006	1.2	1.6	0.3

Per 100,000 population.
Source: National Notifiable Diseases Surveillance System, 1996 to 2006: http://www.cdc.gov/hepatitis/statistics.htm.

the incidence ranging from 5.6 cases for every 100,000 people in the population in 2002 to 2.9 in 2006.

Table 5.6 shows the trend in incidence rates from 1997 to 2006 in the United States for acute viral hepatitis, types A, B, and C (known as non-A, non-B). The rates of all types of hepatitis have significantly decreased, with the greatest decline seen in hepatitis A. This is due in part to improved precautions and awareness.

Prevalence

Prevalence (it is not necessary to use the word *rate* with prevalence because prevalence is a rate) measures the number of people with a disease in the population. Prevalence can be measured at a specific point in time or over a period of time. When you are measuring the total number of cases of a disease occurring in a specified population at a particular point in time, this is the called the point prevalence. The *point prevalence* (usually just called prevalence) is the total number of cases of a disease occurring in a specified population at a particular point in time divided by the total number of people in that population present at that point in time. The (point) prevalence is

$$\frac{\text{number of existing cases of a disease in a specific population at a specific time}}{\text{total number of people in a specific population at a specific time}}$$

Prevalence is used by hospitals and health agencies every day to evaluate the health of the community. For example, hospitals conduct screening programs for people with hypertension who live in the community. An example is a blood pressure screening program that is conducted on the first day of the month with 1,500 people. Of those screened, 150 people have systolic and diastolic blood pressures that indicate that they have hypertension. The prevalence of this screened population is 150 per 1,500, or 10 percent. This indicates that currently 10 percent of the screened population has hypertension. This does not mean that the risk of developing hypertension in the population is 10 percent because prevalence cannot measure risk of getting a disease. Prevalence only provides information about the people at the time of the screening, so the reasons why they developed hypertension cannot be traced, and risk factors cannot be identified. It is important to remember that incidence is what measures the risk in a population.

Table 5.7 presents the results of the 2007 Behavioral Risk Factor Surveillance System (BRFSS) for the prevalence of diabetes in the United States, according to age. The specific question on the survey was, "Have you ever been told by a doctor that you have diabetes?" The prevalence in the United States in 2007 was 9.0 percent, and the older an individual, the greater the prevalence.

The prevalence across age groups shows a significant difference, indicating the relationship between age and diabetes. This increase with age is characteristic of most chronic diseases.[2]

BRFSS

The Behavioral Risk Factor Surveillance System (BRFSS) is a state-based system of health surveys that collects information on health risk behaviors, preventive health practices, and health care access primarily related to chronic disease and injury.

BRFSS was established in 1984 by the Centers for Disease Control and Prevention (CDC). Today, data are collected monthly in all fifty states, the District of Columbia, Puerto Rico, the U.S. Virgin Islands, and Guam. More than 350,000 adults are interviewed each year by telephone. The BRFSS data are used to identify health problems, establish and track health objectives, and develop and evaluate public health policies and programs.

Source: Centers for Disease Control and Prevention, http://www.cdc.gov/brfss.

TABLE 5.7: Prevalence of Diabetes in the United States, 2007, by Age*

Age Group	Yes	No
Overall, years	9.0	91.0
18 to 24	1.6	98.4
25 to 34	3.5	96.5
35 to 44	5.4	94.6
45 to 54	8.8	91.2
55 to 64	14.8	85.2
65 and older	18.8	81.2

*Percent.
Source: Centers for Disease Control and Prevention. *National Vital Statistics Report 56*(10), April 24, 2008.

Table 5.8 presents the prevalence of obesity for selected states in 2007. Mississippi has the highest prevalence of 32.0 percent, with Tennessee the second highest with a prevalence of 30.1 percent. Colorado has the lowest prevalence of 18.7 percent.

When prevalence is measured over a period of time, it is called *period prevalence.* The word "period" is always included to distinguish it from point prevalence. The period prevalence combines the incidence and prevalence rates and is defined as

$$\frac{\text{number of existing cases of a disease population at a specific time plus number of new cases of a disease in a specific population during a specified period}}{\text{total number of people in a specific population during a specified period}}$$

The period prevalence is used for large populations because it is difficult to measure a point in time in large groups of people. Because of the large number of people, prevalence measurement has to be done over a period of time.

What happens with the period prevalence is that the point in time used in the point prevalence is expanded several months or a year. In this new expanded point in time (which becomes a period of time), the percentage of the people in a population with a disease is identified as the period prevalence rate. During this expanded time period, both existing cases (those known at the beginning of the time period) and new cases (those that develop during the time period) are identified. If the time period is a year, then the period prevalence rate is the point prevalence rate at the beginning of the year plus the year's incidence rate.

TABLE 5.8: Prevalence of Obesity in Selected States, 2007*

State	Prevalence	State	Prevalence
Arizona	25.4	New Hampshire	24.4
Arkansas	28.7	New Jersey	23.5
California	22.6	New Mexico	24.0
Colorado	18.7	New York	25.0
Connecticut	21.2	North Carolina	28.0
Delaware	27.4	North Dakota	26.5
Florida	23.6	Ohio	27.5
Georgia	28.2	Oklahoma	28.1
Hawaii	21.4	Oregon	25.5
Idaho	24.5	Pennsylvania	27.1
Iowa	26.9	South Dakota	26.2
Kansas	26.9	Tennessee	30.1
Kentucky	27.4	Texas	28.1
Louisiana	29.8	Utah	21.8
Maine	24.8	Vermont	21.3
Maryland	25.4	Virginia	24.3
Massachusetts	21.3	Washington	25.3
Michigan	27.7	Washington, D.C.	21.8
Minnesota	25.6	West Virginia	29.5
Mississippi	32.0	Wisconsin	24.7
Missouri	27.5	Wyoming	23.7
Nevada	24.1		

*Percent.
Source: Centers for Disease Control and Prevention, Behavioral Risk Factor Surveillance System (BRFSS).

An example of period prevalence is as follows. Suppose that the number of people with diabetes who receive health care on June 30, 2008, at East Bank Regional Hospital, which is the only hospital in a community of 100,000 people, was 75. The prevalence rate on June 30, 2008, of people with diabetes receiving health care was 75 per 100,000. If the number of people with diabetes who received health care at East Bank Regional Hospital between July 1, 2008, and December 31, 2008, was 150, then the incidence rate was 150 people per 100,000. The period prevalence from June 30, 2008, to December 31, 2008, would be 225 people per 100,000.

Figure 5.1 presents the period prevalence of overweight children aged six to eleven years and teenagers aged twelve to nineteen years. The prevalence information is shown in four time periods: 1971 to 1974, 1976 to 1980, 1988 to 1994, and 1999 to 2002. The period prevalence during these times indicates that overweight among children and teenagers more than tripled between the 1960s and 2002.[3]

FIGURE 5.1: Period prevalence of overweight among children and teenagers by age group and selected period, United States, 1971 to 2002

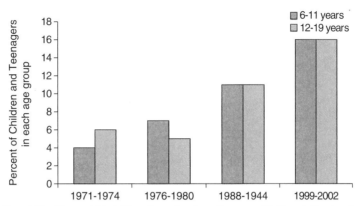

Source: National Health and Nutrition Examination Surveys, National Center for Health Statistics, Centers for Disease Control and Prevention.

Incidence and prevalence are often confused as measuring the same thing, but incidence measures new cases of a disease, and prevalence measures those cases already present in a population. However, incidence is directly related to prevalence. People must first get the disease (become a new case) before they can be included in the prevalence. When they first get the disease and become a new case, they are counted as part of the incidence. So as the incidence increases, the prevalence increases. As the incidence decreases, the prevalence also decreases.

Relationship Between Prevalence and Incidence

Prevalence ≈ Incidence × the time duration of a disease

In addition to incidence, prevalence is also directly affected by how long someone has a disease (known as the duration of a disease). If someone has a disease that has no cure and lasts a long time (for example, diabetes), then the prevalence of that disease will be high. The reason is that there is a greater opportunity to detect this disease at many points in time. So when you are measuring prevalence of this chronic disease, more cases will be found. Conversely, if someone has a disease that does not last long and can be cured (for example, mononucleosis symptoms last only four weeks), the prevalence will be low. Because the disease duration is short, there is less of an opportunity to detect it at any point in time.

Prevalence is affected by both the occurrence of disease (measured by the incidence) and the average duration of disease. As both the incidence rate and duration of disease increase, prevalence experiences an associated increase. If incidence and duration decrease, so does the prevalence.[4]

Mortality

The basic form of a *mortality rate* is

$$\frac{\text{number of deaths in a population during a specified period}}{\text{number of people in a population during a specified period}}$$

The number of deaths in the numerator is obtained from information collected from death certificates. The number of people in the population in the denominator comes from U.S. Census information.

The formula above is known as the overall mortality rate, also called the crude death rate or total death rate, and it measures the frequency of all deaths in a population. Table 5.9 presents the overall crude death rate in the United States, and crude death rates from the fifteen leading causes of death during 2005. The table shows that the total number of deaths equaled 2,488,017, and the mortality rate was 825.9 per 100,000 people in the population. Of these, diseases of the heart made up 652,091 deaths, or 26 percent of the total. Deaths from malignant neoplasms were a close second with 559,312 deaths, or 22.8 percent. The number of people who died from diabetes mellitus was 75,119, or 3.1 percent. These rates measure the frequency of death by the cause of death and are known as the *cause-specific mortality rate*. This rate is defined as follows:

$$\frac{\begin{array}{c}\text{number of deaths due to a specific cause}\\ \text{in a specific population during a specified period}\end{array}}{\text{total number of people in a specific population during a specified period}}$$

As in the total death rate above, the specified period is the same in the numerator and denominator. Again, the sources of information are death certificates for

TABLE 5.9: Number of Deaths and Crude Death Rates* for the 15 Leading Causes of Death, 2005

Cause of Death	Number	Rate
All causes	2,488,017	825.9
Diseases of the heart	652,091	220.0
Malignant neoplasms	559,312	188.7
Cerebrovascular diseases	143,579	48.4
Chronic lower respiratory tract diseases	130,933	44.2
Accidents (unintentional injuries)	117,809	39.7
Diabetes mellitus	75,119	25.3
Alzheimer's disease	71,599	24.2
Influenza and pneumonia	63,001	21.3
Nephritis, nephritic syndrome, and nephrosis	43,901	14.8
Septicemia	34,136	11.5
Intentional Self-harm (suicide)	32,637	11.0
Chronic liver disease and cirrhosis	27,530	9.3
Essential (primary) hypertension and hypertensive liver disease	24,902	8.4
Parkinson's disease	19,544	6.6
Assault (homicide)	18,124	6.1
All other causes	433,800	146.4

*Per 100,000 population.
Source: Centers for Disease Control and Prevention, *National Vital Statistics Report 56*(10), April 24, 2008.

the numerator and the U.S. Census for the denominator. Table 5.10 shows that the cause-specific mortality rate for diseases of the heart (referred to as the heart disease death rate) is the highest at 220.0 deaths per 100,000 people in the population. Diabetes mellitus had a cause-specific mortality rate of 25.3 deaths per 100,000 people in the population.

Table 5.10 shows mortality at different ages. This is known as the *age-specific mortality rate*, and is defined as

$$\frac{\text{number of deaths within a specific age group in a specific population during a specified period of time}}{\text{total number of people in a specific population during a specified period of time}}$$

In general, as age increases, the mortality rate increases. This trend is seen with chronic diseases. The only exceptions are seen in suicide and homicide. It

TABLE 5.10: Cause-Specific Death Rates* by Age for the 15
Leading Causes of Death, United States, 2005,
for Selected Age Categories

Cause of Death	All Ages	5 to 14 Years	15 to 24 Years	25 to 34 Years	45 to 54 Years	55 to 64 Years	65 to 74 Years	75 to 84 Years
All causes	825.9	16.3	81.4	104.4	432.0	906.9	2,137.1	5,260.0
Diseases of the heart	220.0	0.6	2.7	8.1	89.7	214.8	518.9	1,460.8
Malignant neoplasms	188.7	2.5	4.1	9.0	118.6	326.9	742.7	1,274.8
Cerebrovascular diseases	48.4	0.2	0.5	1.4	15.0	33.0	101.1	359.0
Chronic lower respiratory tract diseases	44.2	0.3	0.4	0.6	9.4	42.0	160.5	385.6
Accidents (unintentional injuries)	39.7	6.0	37.4	34.9	43.2	35.8	46.3	106.1
Diabetes mellitus	25.3	0.1	0.5	1.5	13.4	37.2	86.8	177.2
Alzheimer's disease	24.2	—	—	—	0.2	2.1	20.5	177.3
Influenza and pneumonia	21.3	0.3	0.4	0.9	5.1	11.3	35.5	142.2
Nephritis, nephritic syndrome, and nephrosis	14.8	0.1	0.2	0.7	4.8	13.6	39.3	110.3
Septicemia	11.5	0.2	0.4	0.8	5.2	12.9	32.6	81.4
Intentional self-harm (suicide)	11.0	0.7	10.0	12.4	16.5	13.9	12.6	16.9
Chronic liver disease	9.3	—	0.1	0.8	17.7	23.5	27.2	29.0
Essential (primary) hypertension and hypertensive liver disease	8.4	—	0.1	0.2	2.7	6.4	17.7	55.6
Parkinson's disease	6.6				0.2	1.4	13.0	71.2
Assault (homicide)	6.1	0.8	13.0	11.8	4.8	2.8	2.4	2.2

*Per 100,000 population.
Source: Centers for Disease Control and Prevention. *National Vital Statistics Report 56*(10), April 24, 2008.

is also important to notice that the death rate for most causes dramatically increases after age forty-five.

Other Measures of Mortality

The mortality rates shown above are the ones that are commonly reported and reviewed. Several other mortality measures are used to measure the frequency of deaths among mothers and children. The most commonly used measure is the *infant mortality rate*, which is defined as

$$\frac{\text{total number of deaths among people younger}}{\text{total number of live births in a specific population during a specified period}}$$

The source of information in the numerator is death certificates and birth certificates in the denominator.

Other measurements of death in children are the neonatal and postneonatal mortality rates. These rates are subsets of the infant mortality rates because causes of death during the neonatal and post-neonatal periods may be different. The *neonatal mortality rate* is defined as

$$\frac{\text{total number of deaths among people younger}}{\text{total number of live births in a specific population during a specified period}}$$

The neonatal mortality rate measures the frequency of death in infants during the first twenty-eight days of life. Common causes of death during this period include congenital abnormalities, pregnancy-related problems, slow fetal growth, and trauma at birth.

The *postneonatal mortality rate* (age twenty-eight days to eleven months) is defined as

$$\frac{\text{total number of deaths among people between ages 28 days}}{\text{total number of live births minus the total number of}}$$
$$\frac{\text{and 11 months in a specific population during a specified period}}{\text{neonatal deaths in a specific population during a specified period}}$$

The postneonatal mortality rate measures how often infants die after surviving the first twenty-eight days of life. Some causes of death in the first twenty-eight days include environmental causes, including sudden infant death syndrome (SIDS) and accidents.

SUDDEN INFANT DEATH SYNDROME

Sudden infant death syndrome (SIDS) is the unexpected death of an infant younger than one year that remains unexplained after a thorough investigation. Typically the infant is found dead after having been put to bed and exhibits no signs of having suffered.

Each year in the United States, more than 4,500 infants die suddenly of no obvious cause. Half of these sudden unexpected infant deaths (SUID) are due to SIDS, the leading cause of SUID and of all deaths among infants aged one to twelve months.

Source: Centers for Disease Control and Prevention. Sudden Infant Death Syndrome (SIDS) and Sudden Unexpected Infant Death (SUID). http://www.cdc.gov/SIDS/index.htm.

Table 5.11 presents information on infant, neonatal, and postneonatal mortality in the United States in 2005. It is apparent that these rates have not changed over the six-year period. The infant mortality rate has remained the same, and in 2005 it was 6.87 deaths per 1,000 live births. The same is true for both the neonatal mortality rate and the postneonatal mortality rate.

TABLE 5.11: Infant, Neonatal, and Postneonatal Mortality Rates* in the United States, 2000 to 2005

Year	Infant Mortality Rate	Neonatal Mortality Rate	Postneonatal Mortality Rate
2000	6.91	4.63	2.28
2001	6.85	4.54	2.31
2002	6.97	4.66	2.31
2003	6.85	4.62	2.31
2004	6.79	4.52	2.27
2005	6.87	4.54	2.34

*Per 1,000 live births.
Source: Centers for Disease Control and Prevention. *National Vital Statistics Report 56*(10), April 24, 2008.

TABLE 5.12: Infant, Neonatal, and Postneonatal Mortality Rates*
by Race of the Mother in the United States, 2000 to 2005

Year	Infant Mortality Rate	Neonatal Mortality Rate	Postneonatal Mortality Rate
White Mother			
2000	6.21	3.82	1.86
2001	5.65	3.78	1.87
2002	5.79	3.89	1.89
2003	5.72	3.87	1.84
2004	5.66	3.78	1.87
2005	5.73	3.79	1.94
Black Mother			
2000	14.09	9.38	4.70
2001	14.02	9.21	4.81
2002	14.36	9.51	4.85
2003	14.01	9.40	4.60
2004	13.79	9.13	4.66
2005	13.73	9.07	4.67

*Per 1,000 live births.
Source: Centers for Disease Control and Prevention. *National Vital Statistics Report 56*(10), April 24, 2008.

Table 5.12 presents infant, neonatal, and postneonatal mortality rates from 2000 to 2005 in the United States categorized by the race of the mother. Again, the rates have not changed much from 2000 to 2005. But there are significant differences in these rates. The infant mortality rate seen in black mothers is more than two times higher than what is seen in white mothers. This difference is larger between white and black mothers in neonatal and postneonatal mortality rates.

The last mortality rate in child populations is the fetal death rate. The *fetal death rate*, which is also known as the stillborn rate, is defined as

$$\frac{\text{total number of fetal deaths among fetuses of 20 weeks or}}{\text{more gestation in a specific population during a specified period}}$$
$$\frac{}{\text{total number of live births plus fetal deaths}}$$
$$\text{in a specific population during a specified period}$$

Table 5.13 presents information about fetal deaths in the United States from 2000 to 2004. The fetal death rate has been stable since 2000.

There are two other measures of mortality that we must discuss. The first is the *case-fatality rate*, which is

TABLE 5.13: Fetal Death Rates* in the United States, 2000 to 2004

Year	Fetal Death Rate
2000	6.61
2001	6.51
2002	6.41
2003	6.23
2004	6.20

*Rate per 1,000 live births plus fetal deaths.
Source: National Center for Health Statistics. Centers for Disease Control and Prevention, National Vital Statistics System.

$$\frac{\text{number of people with a disease who die of that disease in a specific population during a specified period}}{\text{total number of people with a disease in a specific population during a specified period}}$$

The case-fatality rate is usually a percentage of people with a disease who die as a result of that disease during a specified period. Case-fatality rate is used in disease outbreaks when all patients are observed for an adequate period to include all deaths that can be traced back to that disease. It is also used in hospitals to identify how many patients die while they are in the hospital.

The final mortality measurement that we will discuss is the proportionate mortality ratio. This measure is not a rate but is a special type of ratio called a proportion. Before we define the proportionate mortality ratio, let's discuss the meaning and difference between a ratio and a proportion.

A proportion is a type of ratio with two distinctions. First, the number in the numerator is included in the denominator. Second, proportions are always expressed as a percentage. As with ratios, a unit of time must be expressed in proportions.

The *proportionate mortality ratio*, known as the PMR, is defined as

$$\frac{\text{number of deaths from a specific cause of death in a specific population during a specified period} \times 100}{\text{total number of deaths from all causes in a specific population during a specified period}}$$

TABLE 5.14: PMR for Deaths in Infants Due to the Five Leading
Causes of Death in the United States, 2004*

Cause of Death	Number of Deaths	PMR
All causes	27,936	100.0
Congenital malformations, including chromosomal abnormalities	5,622	20.1
Disorders related to short gestation and low birth weight	4,642	16.6
Sudden infant death syndrome	2,246	8.0
Newborn affected by maternal complications of pregnancy	1,715	6.1
Accidents (unintentional injuries)	1,052	3.8

*PMR is expressed as a percentage. Infants are considered to be younger than one year.
Source: Centers for Disease Control and Prevention. National Vital Statistics Reports 56(5), Nov. 20, 2007.

The PMR indicates what proportion of deaths can be traced to a specific cause. This is similar to the cause-specific mortality rate, except for the difference in the denominator. The denominator of the cause-specific mortality ratio is the total number of people in the population, whereas in the PMR it is the total number of all deaths.

Table 5.14 gives examples of the PMR for five leading causes of death in infants (younger than one year). The highest PMR is seen in deaths caused by congenital malformations, including chromosomal abnormalities. The second highest PMR is death caused by short gestation, which usually results in low birth weight. The third highest is associated with SIDS.

Other Measures

Survival Rates

The survival rate can be thought of as being the opposite of the mortality rate. The survival rate identifies those people who live with a disease. Survival rate is used with diseases that last a long time, as is the case with most chronic diseases (cancers in particular). The survival rate is the percentage of people who live over a specified period, usually five years. In other words, the survival rate tells us the chance that someone will live for a specified period with a chronic disease. The survival rate is defined as

TABLE 5.15: Five-Year Cancer Survival Rates for Selected Cancers by Race, 1987–1989 Through 1996–2003

	1987–1989	1990–1992	1993–1995	1996–2003
Whites				
All cancers	57.7	62.4	63.4	67.0
Oral cavity and pharynx	56.6	58.7	60.9	62.0
Esophagus	11.0	13.6	14.3	17.5
Stomach	19.1	19.3	20.7	22.2
Colon	61.7	63.9	61.4	65.6
Rectum	59.6	61.2	61.7	66.4
Pancreas	3.4	4.6	4.2	4.9
Lung and bronchus	13.8	14.5	15.1	15.7
Blacks				
All cancers	43.6	48.2	52.8	57.0
Oral cavity and pharynx	34.4	33.3	38.2	40.6
Esophagus	6.4	9.4	7.5	10.9
Stomach	20.0	24.1	19.8	24.2
Colon	53.2	54.2	52.3	54.7
Rectum	53.5	52.2	54.8	58.4
Pancreas	5.7	3.7	3.7	4.6
Lung and bronchus	11.2	10.8	13.0	12.5

Source: National Institutes of Health, National Cancer Institute, Surveillance, Epidemiology, and End Results (SEER) Program.

$$\frac{\text{total number of people with a chronic disease who survive over a specified period}}{\text{total number of people with a chronic disease during the same specified period}}$$

Table 5.15 shows five-year cancer survival rates for several cancers by race from 1987 to 2003. Whites have had higher survival rates for all cancers since 1987. This is true for all cancers except stomach cancer.

Immunization Rates

Most childhood diseases are preventable by taking vaccines. The CDC has immunization schedules for children and schedules for keeping information about vaccine coverage. The percentage of children who have received the scheduled immunizations is called the immunization rate.

VACCINE-PREVENTABLE DISEASES

Anthrax, cervical cancer, diphtheria, hepatitis A, *Haemophilus influenzae* type B, human papillomavirus (HPV), influenza (flu), Japanese encephalitis, Lyme disease, measles, meningococcal, monkeypox, mumps, pertussis (whooping cough), pneumococcal, poliomyelitis (polio), rabies, rotavirus, rubella (German measles), shingles (herpes zoster), smallpox, tetanus (lockjaw), tuberculosis, varicella (chickenpox), and yellow fever.

Source: Centers for Disease Control and Prevention. http://www.cdc.gov/vaccines/vpd-vac/default.htm.

The CDC recommends immunization for the following diseases from birth through age six years: hepatitis B, rotavirus, diphtheria, tetanus, pertussis (whooping cough), *Haemophilus influenzae* type b, pneumococcal, poliomyelitis (polio), influenza (flu), measles, mumps, rubella (German measles), varicella (chickenpox), hepatitis A, and meningococcal. The CDC also monitors immunizations.[5] Table 5.16 presents information about immunization coverage from 2000 to 2004.

TABLE 5.16: Estimated Vaccination Coverage (Percentage) Among Children Ages 19 to 35 Months, by Vaccine and Dosage, 2000 to 2004

Vaccine	2000	2001	2002	2003	2004
DTP/DT/DTaP					
3 doses	94.1	94.3	94.9	96.0	95.9
4 doses	81.7	82.1	81.6	84.8	85.5
Poliovirus	89.5	89.4	90.2	91.6	91.6
MMR	90.5	91.4	91.6	93.0	93.5
Hepatitis B	90.3	88.9	89.9	92.4	92.4
Varicella	67.8	76.3	80.6	84.8	87.5
Pneumococcal virus					
3 doses	—	—	40.8	68.1	73.2
4 doses	—	—	—	35.8	43.4

DTP/DT/DTaP = various formulations of diphtheria and tetanus toxoids and pertussis
MMR = measles, mumps, and rubella
Source: Centers for Disease Control and Prevention, http://www.cdc.gov/vaccines/vpd-vac/default.htm.

Fertility Rate

The fertility rate is used to indicate the chance for population growth. It measures the number of children born for every woman in the childbearing years (considered to be from ages fifteen to forty-four). The *fertility rate* is defined as

$$\frac{\text{total number of live births in a specific population during a specified period of time}}{\text{total number of females between the ages of 15 to 44 years in a specific population during a specified period of time}}$$

Table 5.17 shows total fertility rates for selected countries. The highest fertility rate is seen in Mali. High fertility rates are seen in developing countries, and lower rates are seen in developed countries like the United States, which has a fertility rate of 2.1.

TABLE 5.17: Estimated Fertility Rates in Selected Countries, 2008*

Country	Fertility Rate
Mali	7.34
Afghanistan	6.58
Kenya	4.70
Iraq	3.97
Pakistan	3.58
Honduras	3.38
Dominican Republic	2.78
Israel	2.77
India	2.72
Peru	2.42
United States	2.10
France	1.98
Ireland	1.85
Norway	1.78
Australia	1.76
Sweden	1.67
United Kingdom	1.66
Canada	1.57
Italy	1.30
Japan	1.22

*Rate of births per woman between the ages of 15 and 44 years.
Source: CIA. *World Fact Book,* 2008.

Health Status

The health status of a population can be described in various ways because there is no one acceptable measure. Commonly used epidemiological measures have been accepted as indicating the health of a population. These measures are mortality, morbidity, communicable disease rates, occupational injury, and illness rates. The CDC uses self-reported health status and limitation in activity caused by a person's health as a way to describe health status.[6]

Table 5.18 presents information from a self-reported health status assessment. The table shows that most people between the ages of eighteen and forty-four feel that their health is better than fair to poor. More than 30 percent of people older than seventy-five years report that their health is fair to poor. Slightly more women (9.5 percent) reported that their health was fair to poor than men (9.0 percent). Whites reported the best health, with only 8.6 percent indicating that their health was fair to poor. More than 14 percent of blacks reported fair to poor health, closely followed by Hispanics or Latinos.

TABLE 5.18: Self-Assessed Health Status, Poor or Fair, by Age, Sex, and Race in the United States, 2002 to 2006*

	2003	2004	2005	2006
Overall	9.2	9.3	9.2	9.2
Age, years				
Younger than 18	1.8	1.8	1.8	1.9
18 to 44	5.6	5.7	5.5	5.7
45 to 54	12.1	12.3	11.6	12.9
55 to 64	18.9	17.9	18.3	18.8
65 and older	25.5	26.7	26.6	24.8
Sex				
Male	8.8	9.0	8.8	9.0
Female	9.5	9.6	9.5	9.5
Race				
White	8.5	8.6	8.6	8.6
Black	14.7	14.6	14.3	14.4
Hispanic or Latino	13.9	13.3	13.3	13.0
Asian	7.4	8.6	6.8	6.9
American Indian or Alaska Native	16.3	16.5	13.2	12.1

*Percentage of persons with fair or poor health.
Source: Centers for Disease Control and Prevention, National Center for Health Statistics, http://apps.nccd.cdc.gov/HRQOL.

TABLE 5.19: Potential Years of Life Lost (PYLL) Before Age 75,
United States, 2005

Cause of Death	PYLL	Percentage
All Causes	20,431,940	100.0
Malignant neoplasms	4,323,414	21.2
Unintentional injury	3,148,925	15.4
Heart disease	3,117,388	15.3
Perinatal period	1,089,395	5.3
Suicide	964,532	4.7
Homicide	770,798	3.8
Congenital anomalies	577,246	2.8
Cerebrovascular	533,900	2.6
Diabetes mellitus	507,621	2.5
Chronic low respiratory tract disease	492,913	2.4
All others	4,905,808	24.0

Source: Centers for Disease Control and Prevention, National Center for Injury Prevention and Control, http://www.cdc.gov/nchs/hus.htm.

Potential Years of Life Lost

When people die before it is expected, in addition to emotional and family concerns, society misses out on the contributions they would have made had they lived a full life. There is an epidemiology measurement that tries to explain the impact of these lost years of life. *Potential years of life lost* (PYLL) is used as an indication of premature death and represents the number of years that are lost because someone dies earlier than expected. PYLL uses premature death to mean when someone does not live until they reach age seventy-five years. Any death between ages zero and seventy-four is considered premature.[7]

The PYLL is calculated in a manner that assigns more importance to deaths that occur at younger than older ages. The PYLL uses seventy-five years as a point of reference, so people who die after age seventy-five are not included in the calculation. Table 5.19 presents information on PYLL, which is calculated by dividing the total number of potential years of life lost by the total number of people in the population who are younger than seventy-five years.

Graphing Health and Disease Measurements

Types of Graphs

Graphs are used to depict health and disease measurements in a way that they are easily understood. Histograms, bar graphs, and pie charts will be discussed.

FIGURE 5.2: Prevalence of diabetes in the United States, 2007, by age

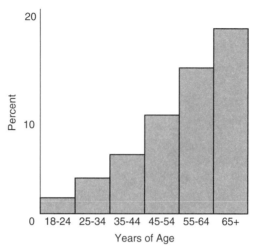

Source: Centers for Disease Control and Prevention, National Vital Statistics report, Volume 56, Number 10, April 24, 2008.

A *histogram* is defined by *Merriam-Webster's Online Dictionary* as "a representation of a frequency distribution by means of rectangles whose widths represent class intervals and whose areas are proportional to the corresponding frequencies." A *frequency distribution* is a table that presents the values of the health and disease measurements.

The histogram graphs numbers according to how often they appear in the data. Histograms compare two sets of data, and from the visual presentation conclusions may be drawn about any differences. Figure 5.2 presents a histogram that shows the prevalence of diabetes in the United States in 2007. It is easy to see that diabetes prevalence increases with age, which is expected because diabetes is a chronic disease. The benefit of histograms is that large amounts of information can be easily evaluated by the construction of one graph that shows peaks in the data.

The second graph type is the *bar graph.* Bar graphs are most often used to compare what is called qualitative variables, such as different hospitals. The difference between bar graphs and histograms is that the bars in histograms represent a range of values rather than a single value as in a bar graph. An example of a bar graph is as follows: using Table 5.1, "AIDS Rates in the United States in 2006 by Race or Ethnic Group," a bar graph can be drawn and is

FIGURE 5.3: AIDS rates by race or ethnic group,
United States, 2006

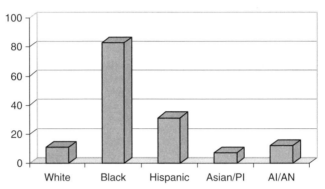

Source: Center for Disease Control and Prevention, National Vital Statistics report, Volume 56, Number 10, April 24, 2008.

FIGURE 5.4: Case-fatality rates for stroke per 100 people admitted to a hospital

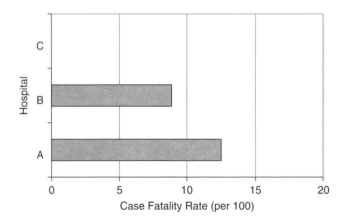

shown in Figure 5.3. The graph is easy to construct and can be used to explain the disease measurement. In Figure 5.3 it is easy to see that the AIDS rate for African Americans is significantly higher than for other races or ethnic groups.

Bar graphs can also be shown as horizontal depictions of information. Figure 5.4 shows a horizontal bar graph of case-fatality rates (per 100 people in the population) from stroke for three hospitals, which are labeled Hospital A, B, and

FIGURE 5.5: Infant mortality and neonatal and postneonatal deaths in the United States, 2005

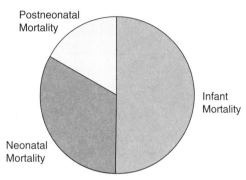

Source: National Vital Statistics report, Volume 56, Number 10, April 24, 2008. Centers for Disease Control and Prevention.

C. The bars of the graph indicate which hospital has the highest case-fatality rate.

The next type of graph is called a *pie chart.* Pie charts present information in the form of pie slices. The pie slices show the relative difference of the information by each group. Each slice of the pie represents the percentage of the frequency distribution. Pie charts are used when the data have a small number of categories. Figure 5.5 shows the number of infant, neonatal, and postneonatal deaths in the United States in 2005.

In summary, histograms should be used when large data sets need to be organized, explained, and communicated to others. Bar graphs should be used to compare information between different groups or to evaluate changes over time. Pie charts are used to compare parts of a data set with the whole, but they do not show changes over time.

Confounding

Up to this point, we have presented and discussed crude rates of disease. These rates were calculated by dividing the number of people with a disease (or the number of deaths) by different denominators (usually the total number of people in the population). So crude rates are based on the actual number of events in a specific population during a specific period.

Crude rates present a problem. Because the denominator is all the people in a population, we do not know the age, race, or sex of the people in the population. As we saw above, many diseases are affected by age, race, or sex. Different populations are made up of very different people. Some populations have a majority of whites whereas others have a majority of blacks. The point is that populations may differ due to differing characteristics, all of which affect the rate of disease. Because we primarily use rates to compare populations, these differences can cause us to make incorrect conclusions from comparisons. Before comparisons can be made, it is important to understand whether the populations are different or the same according to their characteristics.

When we make comparisons of populations that are different in age, sex, race, and the like and the results are inaccurate, it is said to be due to confounding. Confounding is defined as the process of mixing up or lumping together indiscriminately.[8] If confounding exists, then the evaluation of differences between two population groups can be misleading and inaccurate. Any characteristic (or factor) that confounds our comparisons is called a confounding factor and can be defined as (1) a true factor that can cause the disease being compared, and (2) unequally distributed in the populations we are comparing. Unequal distribution means that the populations are different in the amount of each factor: one population has more older people than another, or one population has more African Americans than another population.

The effect of confounding can be eliminated, allowing accurate comparisons to be made in three ways: stratification, matching, and standardization. *Stratification* is a method that separates population information into strata that are defined by the specific confounding factors (for example, by age categories). This will result in equalizing age in the populations that are to be compared, so one of the necessary properties for confounding is eliminated. *Matching* consists of selecting people who have similar characteristics (same age category, same sex, same race) in each population. In other words, people are "matched" according to the possible confounding factor. Again, matching equalizes the distribution of a possible confounding factor. *Standardization* is a process in which crude rates are adjusted by the use of a standard population that equalizes the possible confounding factor in each population. If age is the possible confounding factor, then standardization produces age-adjusted rates.

Two methods of standardization are commonly used. The direct method of standardization develops an adjusted rate that can be used to directly compare the populations. The indirect method does not resulted in an adjusted rate but produces a standardized ratio that can be used to make indirect comparisons. The standardized ratio, which is called the SMR, with the M standing for either morbidity or mortality (depending on whether it is measuring illness or death),

TABLE 5.20: Age-Adjusted Invasive Cancer Incidence Rates by
Primary Site and Race and Ethnicity in the United States, 2004*

Cancer Type	All Races	Whites	Blacks	Hispanics
All sites	537.6	527.7	607.3	415.5
Oral cavity and pharynx	15.7	15.5	17.6	10.4
Digestive tract	105.3	101.6	131.2	104.3
Respiratory tract	93.7	92.4	117.6	55.4
Bones and joints	1.0	1.0	0.9	0.8
Soft tissue including heart	3.6	3.6	3.3	3.3
Skin excluding basal and squamous	23.4	25.4	2.0	5.2
Male genital tract	151.6	141.5	219.7	126.9
Breast	1.4	1.4	1.8	0.9
Urinary tract	57.7	59.7	39.0	38.9
Eye and orbit	0.9	1.0	0.3	0.6
Brain and other nervous system	7.8	8.3	4.5	6.1
Endocrine system	5.4	5.6	3.3	4.2
Lymphomas	25.7	26.2	19.4	22.6
Myeloma	6.8	6.2	13.1	6.4
Leukemias	15.2	15.4	11.8	10.8
Mesothelioma	2.0	2.1	1.1	1.4
Kaposi's sarcoma	0.8	0.7	1.6	1.6
Miscellaneous	19.7	19.7	19.3	15.7

*Rates per 100,000 population.
Source: U.S. Cancer Statistics Working Group, Centers for Disease Control and
Prevention and National Cancer Institute; 2007.

compares each population directly with a standard population and then makes
indirect evaluations of each population. Both types of standardization methods
eliminate the effect of confounding factors.

Table 5.20 presents age-adjusted invasive cancer incidence rates by the
primary site and by race and ethnic group. The incidence rate for all sites is
highest in African Americans, with an age-adjusted rate of 607.3 per 100,000
people in the population. This is also higher than the incidence rate of all races.

Table 5.21 presents crude and age-adjusted death rates for alcohol-induced
causes by race in the United States from 1999 to 2005. The crude and age-
adjusted rates have remained almost the same for all races. But crude rates have
increased for whites (from 7.0 per 100,000 population in 1999 to 7.7 in 2005),
along with a slight increase in age-adjusted rates. Blacks have experienced a
decrease in both crude and age-adjusted rates. The decline in crude rates was
from 7.8 per 100,000 population in 1999 to 5.9 per 100,000 population in 2005.

TABLE 5.21: Crude and Age-Adjusted Death Rates* for Alcohol-Induced Causes, by Race, United States, 1999 to 2005

Year	All Races	White	Black
Crude rates			
1999	7.0	7.0	7.8
2000	7.0	7.1	7.4
2001	7.1	7.2	7.3
2002	7.0	7.2	6.4
2003	7.1	7.4	6.3
2004	7.2	7.5	6.1
2005	7.3	7.7	5.9
Age-adjusted rates			
1999	7.1	6.8	9.8
2000	7.0	6.9	9.1
2001	7.0	6.9	8.9
2002	6.9	6.9	7.8
2003	7.0	7.0	7.4
2004	7.0	7.1	7.2
2005	7.0	7.2	6.8

*Rates per 100,000 population.
Source: Centers for Disease Control and Prevention. *National Vital Statistics Report 56*(10), April 24, 2008.

The decrease in age-adjusted rates was more dramatic, from 9.8 per 100,000 in 1999 to 6.8 per 100,000 in 2005.

Summary

In this chapter we discussed epidemiological measurements, how they are used, and how they are presented for interpretation. There are three basic types of measurements: counts, rates, and ratios. These measurements are used to identify the frequency of health, disease, and death in a population. Rates are the most commonly used epidemiological measurement, and they provide the most information. Disease rates include incidence and prevalence. Death frequency is expressed by several mortality rates and potential years of life lost.

Epidemiological measurements can be graphically presented using histograms, bar graphs, and pie charts. These graphic representations are used to communicate the information contained in the epidemiological measurements.

The notion of confounding was introduced. Confounding can cause errors in the interpretation of comparisons of death and disease between populations.

Several methods exist than can eliminate confounding and better ensure accurate comparisons.

Key Terms

Chapter Exercises

1. Discuss the difference between incidence and prevalence.
2. What information is provided by the Behavioral Risk Factor Surveillance System?
3. What is the difference between the proportionate mortality ratio and other ratios?

Chapter Review

1. Select the rate that best describes the statements below.
   a. Death occurred in 20 percent of the cases of acute myocardial infarction at East Bank Hospital.

    b. Twenty people die each year in the United States for every 1,000 people in the population.

    c. Twenty-five percent of the deaths this year were in people who had heart disease.

    d. Today 15 percent of the people in East Bank County have asthma.

    e. Last year there were 1,500 new cases of HIV infection in East Bank City.

2. The prevalence rate of a disease is the function of

    a. the average duration of the disease.

    b. the incidence rate of the disease.

    c. how quickly people die.

    d. how quickly people are cured.

    e. all of the above.

3. The case-fatality rate is the

    a. number of deaths in a year divided by the total population.

    b. number of deaths from a disease in a specific period divided by the number of people with the disease.

    c. number of new cases of a disease divided by the total population at risk.

    d. number of deaths from a particular disease divided by the total number of deaths.

4. The crude death rate is the

    a. number of deaths in a year divided by the total population.

    b. number of deaths from a disease in a specific period of time divided by the number of people with the disease.

    c. number of new cases of a disease divided by the total population at risk.

    d. number of deaths from a particular disease divided by the total number of deaths.

    e. number of deaths from a particular disease divided by the total population.

5. The cause-specific mortality rate is the

    a. number of deaths in a year divided by the total population.

    b. number of deaths from a disease in a specific period of time divided by the number of people with the disease.

    c. number of new cases of a disease divided by the total population at risk.

    d. number of deaths from a particular disease divided by the total number of deaths.

    e. number of deaths from a particular disease divided by the total population.

6. The incidence rate is the

    a. number of deaths in a year divided by the total population.

b. number of deaths from a disease in a specific period of time divided by the number of people with the disease.

c. number of new cases of a disease divided by the total population at risk.

d. number of deaths from a particular disease divided by the total number of deaths.

e. number of deaths from a particular disease divided by the total population.

7. The proportionate mortality ratio (PMR) is the

a. number of deaths in a year divided by the total population.

b. number of deaths from a disease in a specific period of time divided by the number of people with the disease.

c. number of new cases of a disease divided by the total population at risk.

d. number of deaths from a particular disease divided by the total number of deaths.

e. number of deaths from a particular disease divided by the total population.

8. This measure estimates the risk of developing tuberculosis in your state each year:

a. the incidence rate

b. the point prevalence rate

c. the period prevalence rate

d. none of the above

9. When a true factor of a disease is unequally distributed in two populations, this factor is

a. an artifact.

b. a confounding factor.

c. not a concern.

d. none of the above.

10. Which of the following is used as a denominator for a disease rate?

a. number of cases of disease.

b. number of new cases of disease.

c. persons lost to follow-up.

d. total population.

e. all of the above.

CHAPTER 6

EPIDEMIOLOGY STUDY DESIGNS: OBSERVATIONAL AND EXPERIMENTAL STUDIES

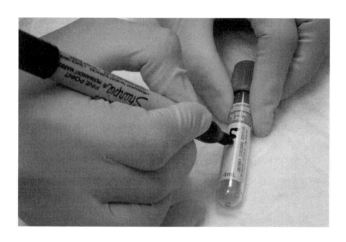

LEARNING OBJECTIVES

On completing this chapter, you will be able to

Describe observational studies
Describe experimental studies
Contrast observational and experimental studies
Describe descriptive study designs
Describe analytical study designs
Describe a randomized clinical trial
Discuss the concepts of bias and validity

Definition of Observational Studies

An *observational study design* is one in which people are observed to see whether a relationship exists between a risk factor and a disease. The observational study design is the most commonly used design in epidemiology. Its major characteristic is that the study design does not affect the outcome, it only observes what happens. In other words, people are not given any treatment or drug; they are simply observed.

During the observation, people are grouped by whether or not they have been exposed to the risk factor. The exposure to the risk factor is not affected by the study but is a personal characteristic. For example, current smokers and nonsmokers are categorized into two groups, and what is observed is whether the disease occurs in both groups. No one is encouraged to smoke or to stop smoking.

Framework and Types of Observational Studies

The framework of observational study designs is presented in Figure 6.1. Descriptive studies collect information that describes disease according to person, place, and time; they are used to determine rates of health and disease. Descriptive studies include ecological studies, case studies, and cross-sectional studies. *Ecological studies* collect information in distinct populations living in specific geographical areas. *Cross-sectional studies* measure the prevalence rate and are concerned with the presence or absence of disease at the present time. *Analytical studies* support hypotheses that exposure to a risk factor is related to the development of a disease. Analytical studies include prospective and retrospective

FIGURE 6.1: Framework of observational studies

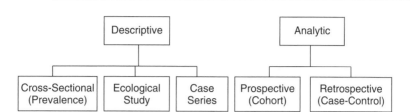

designs. *Retrospective studies,* also known as case-control studies, look at the presence or absence of disease in the past. *Prospective studies,* called cohort studies, follow study groups into the future to observe the presence or absence of disease.

Descriptive Studies

Descriptive studies can be either prospective (studying future events) or retrospective (studying events in the past). These studies evaluate many different types of information, including demographics and morbidity and mortality data. Examples of prospective descriptive study designs include disease registries, mortality data collection, and morbidity data collection. Retrospective descriptive study designs record past measurements of information; included in this category is the U.S. Census and a review of other routinely collected data, such as the Medicare Provider Analysis and Review data file published by the Centers for Medicare and Medicaid Services.

MEDICARE AND MEDICAID

The *Centers for Medicare and Medicaid Services (CMS),* previously known as the *Health Care Financing Administration,* is a federal agency within the U.S. Department of Health and Human Services that administers the Medicare program and works in partnership with state governments to administer Medicaid, the State Children's Health Insurance Program, and health insurance portability standards. In addition to these programs, CMS has other responsibilities, including the administrative simplification standards from the Health Insurance Portability and Accountability Act of 1996, quality standards in long-term care facilities (more commonly referred to as nursing homes) through its survey and certification process, and clinical laboratory quality standards under the Clinical Laboratory Improvement Amendments.

Continued

The *Medicare Provider Analysis and Review (MEDPAR) File* contains data from claims for services provided to beneficiaries admitted to Medicare-certified inpatient hospitals and skilled nursing facilities. The MEDPAR file allows researchers to track inpatient history and patterns or outcomes of care over time.

Source: Department of Health and Human Services, Centers for Medicare and Medicaid Services: http://www.cms.hhs.gov/IdentifiableDataFiles/05_Medicare ProviderAnalysisandReviewFile.asp.

Descriptive studies are not useful for establishing cause-and-effect relationships between risk factors and diseases. But these inexpensive descriptive studies are useful for gathering information that can be used to formulate hypotheses. An example of this is the use of U.S. Census information. If the census data indicate a higher percentage of people older than sixty-five years in a population than what is typical, then a hypothesis can be formulated that this population has a higher death rate than is expected.

There are four specific types of descriptive studies. These are case series, case reports, cross-sectional studies, and ecological studies.

Case Series

A *case series* is a descriptive observational study that evaluates a series of cases of a disease. The purpose of a case series study is to review and describe the clinical signs, disease progression, and disease prognosis. Case series are helpful when you are attempting to formulate hypotheses to be tested using analytical studies. Case series in themselves cannot be used to test hypotheses because only people with the disease are evaluated and there is no comparison group. Case series lack a group of healthy people who are necessary for comparisons.

Case Reports

A *case report* is the description of a single case of a disease. The case report includes the description of the disease manifestations, clinical course, and prognosis. Because it reports a single case, a case report does not provide enough useful information to compare cases of the disease. But case reports are useful in describing how other people have diagnosed and treated a disease as well as the clinical signs after treatment.

Cross-Sectional Study

Cross-sectional studies, also known as prevalence studies, are a type of descriptive study that evaluates the relationship between diseases and risk factors at a specific point in time and in a defined population. Cross-sectional studies are designed to measure the amount of disease in a population, which is the prevalence. In addition, cross-sectional studies measure the amount of a risk factor in a population.

Cross-sectional studies are done in specific geographically defined populations. This study design results in descriptive data showing the pattern of disease and the pattern of risk factors in a population at a specific point.

Cross-sectional studies usually divide the population into two groups of people: those who have been exposed and those who have not been exposed to a risk factor. At the same time, the presence of disease is evaluated in both groups of people. Cross-sectional studies do not allow for establishing cause-and-effect relationships. This is because the current exposure to a risk factor may not be related to the current disease (the disease may be related to exposure to an earlier risk factor). Also, other important prior experiences that may have influenced the disease usually are not known.

Cross-sectional studies are useful because they provide estimates of the extent of a health problem (that is, they provide the prevalence in the population). They can be performed in a relatively short period of time, and large populations can be studied easily. Figure 6.2 presents a graphic representation of the method used in a cross-sectional study.

FIGURE 6.2: Cross-sectional study

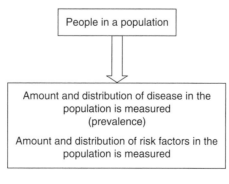

An example of a cross-sectional study is one in which the amount of walking and biking in urban and suburban locations was observed. In this study, the prevalence rate of active commuting to schools was measured, revealing that only 5.0 percent of the study subjects participated in active commuting.[1]

Ecological Study

Ecological studies look at populations of people or groups of people. Ecological studies can be defined as the investigation of the distribution of health and health determinants in groups of people. Ecological studies do not allow for the testing of hypotheses about the relationship between a risk factor and a disease. The time frame for an ecological study is a point in time across a population (you will see that this is also used in cross-sectional studies). Ecological studies investigate the characteristics of a disease in an entire population. The main purpose of ecological studies is descriptive to generate hypotheses.

An example of an ecological study is the evaluation of the relationship between neurobehavioral diseases and contaminants in drinking water. A particular study investigated the relationship between the chemical perchlorate in the drinking water and the prevalence of thyroid diseases and thyroid cancer. The study was conducted in counties in Nevada where contamination of the drinking water with perchlorate had been previously reported.[2]

Why would you choose to do an ecological study? There are several good reasons. First, if information is not available on individual people in the population, then ecological studies are needed to evaluate the entire population. Second, ecological studies are done when personal information is not known, but group data are available. Third, ecological studies are done when large populations (for example, two or more countries) are to be compared.

When ecological studies are done, they usually use measurements that combine several characteristics of the population or groups in the population. Examples of population measurements are average yearly income, the percentage of families living below the federal poverty line, and average number of people living in a household. Group measurements include maximum daily exposure to ozone, average yearly exposure to radon gas, and daily average levels of tobacco smoke in public buildings.

Another example of an ecological study evaluated four sexually transmitted diseases (STDs) in different geographical areas. The study investigated cases of syphilis, gonorrhea, chlamydial infection, and genital herpes in a large county that has both urban and rural areas. These STDs were geocoded by U.S. Census tracts. The information from this study was used to begin geographically specific interventions for these diseases.[3]

STDS

Sexually transmitted diseases are infections that are transmitted by sex with an infected person. STDs are caused by bacteria, parasites, and viruses. STDs include chlamydia, gonorrhea, herpes simplex, HIV/AIDS, human papilloma virus infection, syphilis, and trichomoniasis.

Most STDs affect both men and women, but often they are more severe in women. If a pregnant woman has an STD, the infection can harm the baby.

Source: U.S. National Library of Medicine, http://www.nlm.nih.gov/medlineplus/sexuallytransmitteddiseases.html.

GEOCODING

Geocoding is the process of finding geographical coordinates (latitude and longitude) from other geographical data, such as street addresses or zip codes. Geocoding allows for precise location of cases of diseases. An example is the use of geocoding to identify hospice use by people who later died of cancer.

Source: Porter DE, Kirtland KA, Neet MJ, Williams JL, Ainsworth BE. Consideration for using a geographic information system to access environmental supports for physical activity. *Prevention of Chronic Diseases,* 2004. http://www.cdc.gov/pcd/issues/2004/oct/04_0047.htm.

Analytical Studies

The objective of an analytical study is to establish relationships between risk factors and diseases. In analytical studies, the hypotheses about the relationship between risk factors and diseases are tested by statistical procedures. Analytical studies usually compare two or more groups of people. Prospective studies, known as cohort studies, and retrospective studies, known as case-control studies, are types of analytical epidemiological studies. The term *cohort* has been defined as any group of people who are related in some way or who have experienced the same life events within a selected period of time.

Prospective Study

Prospective or cohort studies are conducted in a forward time manner. That is, people who do not have a disease are identified at the beginning of the prospective study, and they are evaluated into the future for a predetermined period (six months, one year, five years) for the development of a disease. Prospective studies are also often called *longitudinal studies* because they begin at a specified starting point in time and end at some predetermined future time.

The people in the study are divided into two groups: those who have been exposed and those who have not been exposed to a risk factor. People in both groups are evaluated for the development of a disease. Because you are looking for new cases during the study time period, prospective studies measure the *incidence rate*. It is important to remember that in prospective studies, the same method used in evaluating and measuring new cases (the incidence rate) is used in both groups of people. The incidence rate is measured in the group of people who have been exposed to the risk factor and compared with that in the group of people who have not been exposed. In other words, prospective studies are concerned with the frequency of disease in the exposed and nonexposed groups. Figure 6.3 shows the framework of a prospective study.

Prospective studies have distinct advantages over other study designs. Because they start by recording the health of people in both groups, they provide complete information about a person's exposure to a risk factor and a concise view of the time sequence between exposure to a risk factor and the development of a disease. The greatest advantage of prospective studies is that they measure incidence rates. Incidence rates are the best way to evaluate the relationship between exposure to a risk factor and the development of a disease.

FIGURE 6.3: Prospective study

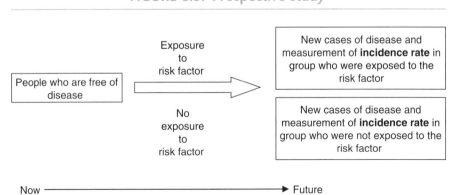

Prospective studies do have some disadvantages. They are not useful for the study of diseases that rarely are seen in the population. It would take a long time to measure the incidence rate because new cases develop so slowly. Prospective studies are not useful when studying disease in which there is a long period between exposure to a risk factor and the resulting development of a disease. Prospective studies are expensive to do because a large number of people must be evaluated periodically over a long period of time.

The Amsterdam Cohort Study on HIV Infection and AIDS is an example of a prospective or cohort study. The study was started in 1984 and continues today. The study evaluates the health of homosexual men every three to six months and includes blood tests. Since 1984 the incidence of HIV infection has decreased significantly from 8 cases per 100 person-years to 1.8 cases per 100 person-years.[4]

Another example of a cohort study is the evaluation of the effect of blood donations in lowering body iron concentrations, which then may cause heart attacks. This study reviewed adults who had donated one unit of blood from 1988 to 1990 and lived in the same city. Information was obtained about the occurrence of acute myocardial infarction, coronary angioplasty, coronary bypass surgery, and death from 1990 to 2000, using hospital records. The study found that the risk of heart attacks and other cardiovascular events was lower in people who donated one unit of blood.[5]

Retrospective Study

Retrospective studies are conducted in a reverse time manner. This means that they use information that has already been collected (called *secondary data*). Secondary data are information that has been collected in the past. Retrospective studies are also called *case-control studies* because the people in the study are divided into two groups: *cases* (have the disease when the study begins) and *controls* (do not have the disease when the study begins). Previously collected information, or information about experiences in the past, about whether the people in each group were exposed to a risk factor is evaluated. The past exposure to a risk factor or factors is determined by reviewing historical data (for example, medical records) and by interviewing study subjects. Figure 6.4 shows the framework of a retrospective study.

Retrospective studies are usually done with small groups of people. The main advantage of retrospective studies is that they are inexpensive to conduct because they use a small number of people and there is no need to observe the study subjects over time into the future. At the beginning of the study, the disease status of the people is identified, then previously collected information and often

FIGURE 6.4: Retrospective study

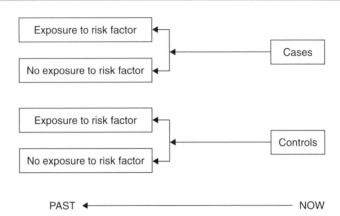

interviews of the study subjects are evaluated to determine who was exposed to the risk factor in the past.

Because there is no follow-up of people in the study, another advantage is that retrospective studies can be performed quickly. The final advantage is that they are useful when studying rarely occurring diseases. Because retrospective studies identify people with a disease when the study begins, it is easy to find an adequate number of cases.

Retrospective studies have three disadvantages. First, they are done on a small number of people, and this makes it difficult to use study results to describe what is happening in the total population. A large number of people are needed in a study to be able to make statements about the meaning of the results for the entire population. Second, because information from interviews of the study subjects is used, there is a greater chance for *bias*. People may not accurately remember if they were exposed to a risk factor in the past (called *recall bias*). The final disadvantage is that because retrospective studies do not identify new cases of a disease, they do not measure incidence rates.

The framework of a retrospective study is the identification of people with a disease (cases) and people without a disease (controls). This can be accomplished by reviewing medical records. The past history of exposure to a risk factor is usually discovered by interviewing study subjects in both groups. The use of and method to obtain information about exposure to a risk factor are accomplished in the same manner for both groups. Retrospective studies are concerned with the frequency and amount of risk factor exposure in cases and controls.

An example of a retrospective study is an investigation of racial and ethnic disparities in diabetes readmissions to hospitals. The relationship between race and ethnicity and hospital readmissions for diabetes-related conditions was evaluated using information obtained from the State Inpatient Databases of the Healthcare Cost and Utilization Project. This database contained information on patients with Medicare, Medicaid, or private insurance who were hospitalized for diabetes-related conditions in a five-state area. The study found that the risk of readmission was significantly lower for whites than for Hispanics and African Americans. This difference was most evident when people were readmitted 180 days after their initial discharge.[6]

Retrospective studies are often done to examine the amount and distribution of a risk factor in a population. One study looked at smoking behaviors in six communities in a large city. A health survey was used to obtain information about the number of people currently smoking, smoking history, and smoking-cessation attempts. The study found that the smoking prevalence rate was 18 percent in the wealthy community that was predominantly white and 39 percent in the poorest, predominantly black, community. It was also discovered that men in the poorest community who live in households without telephones were more likely to smoke.[7]

Examples of Observational Studies

One example of an observational study involves a cross-sectional study at a large manufacturing company that became concerned with absenteeism and declining work productivity.[8] The company decided to implement a wellness program at the factory for its employees. A needs assessment and baseline health data were needed before the company could implement the program. A local hospital took histories and conducted physical examinations and cholesterol screening for the company's 2,500 employees. Of the total number of people who were examined, 1,701 were male employees. Results of these examinations included prevalence estimates on smoking habits, obesity, dietary habits, exercise, abnormal levels of low-density lipoproteins (LDL cholesterol, which is the harmful form of cholesterol), and other employee characteristics. Specifically, the study found that the amount of high-density lipoproteins (HDL cholesterol, which is the good form of cholesterol) is reduced in people with a high BMI, in people who smoke, and in people who have a high body fat percentage. This information had two purposes. First, information about the prevalence of risk factors can be used for proper planning of wellness programs (for example, weight reduction, smoking cessation, and so on). Second, the health effects of the wellness program could be determined by comparing baseline health status data with future wellness program data.

A second example of a cross-sectional study is the Harvard School of Public Health College Alcohol Study, which has been conducted at different times since 1993.[9] In 1999 the study surveyed more than 14,000 college students in 119 four-year colleges in 39 states by mailed questionnaires. The results indicated that 44 percent of college students were binge drinkers of alcohol. These binge drinkers were more likely to experience alcohol-related problems.

The Harvard School of Public Health College Alcohol Study learned the following: there is a need to lower drinking thresholds, there are harmful effects on other students and neighbors, the binge-drinking problem continues to grow, and the college environment has an influence on the amount of drinking by students. The study also found that there is less drinking among college students in states that have more restrictions on underage drinking and sales of alcoholic beverages as well as more resources allocated to enforcing drunk-driving laws.[10]

Comparison of Observational Studies

Figure 6.5 presents a comparison of observational studies according to the study characteristics, time (orientation and duration), follow-up, and relative cost. This summary figure shows that the most expensive study design is the prospective study, but it may provide the best information because it determines the incidence rate of a disease. The retrospective study is inexpensive and quick, but its results may be biased. The case series, cross-sectional, and ecological studies provide useful information, are quick and inexpensive, but their results cannot be used to test hypotheses about the relationship between risk factors and diseases. Figure 6.5 tells us that there is no one perfect study design. The several study designs exist because of the need to gather information in different ways when it is needed.

Definition of Experimental Studies

Experimental studies have a distinct difference from observational studies. In experimental studies, the investigator can manipulate (by either introducing or altering the amount of) one or more risk factors for a disease. In addition, external factors can be controlled to eliminate their effect. Because of the nature of experimental studies, they provide strong evidence for the testing of study hypotheses. However, they are expensive and difficult to conduct.

FIGURE 6.5: Comparison of observational studies

Study	Characteristics	Time Orientation	Time Duration	Follow-up	Cost
Case Series	Group of cases, no controls	Present	Quick		Inexpensive
Cross-sectional	Point-in-time evaluation; **prevalence rate** measurement is result	Present	Quick	None	Inexpensive
Ecological	Study by geographic area	Present	Quick	None	Inexpensive
Prospective	One group is exposed and the other group is not exposed to a risk factor; **incidence rate** measurement is result	Future	Very time consuming	For a period of time into the future	Expensive
Retrospective	One group has a disease and the other group does not have a disease	Present	Quick	None	Inexpensive

Framework and Types of Experimental Studies

The framework of an experimental study consists of the researcher(s) selecting a number of people who are similar in some characteristics. The people in the experimental study need to be similar (same age, same sex, same race, from the same neighborhood, same socioeconomic group) so that the effect of confounding is minimized. The researcher then randomly selects and divides these people into subgroups. These subgroups are called the experimental and control groups. The experimental group is given a risk factor for a disease. Both experimental and control groups are observed for the development of the disease. Pure experimental studies are no longer done because of the ethical considerations of giving

FIGURE 6.6: Experimental studies

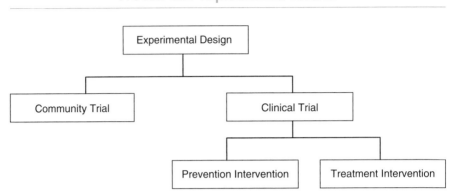

people a risk factor that may be associated with a disease. In addition, experimental studies are expensive to conduct. The only type of experimental study that is done today is the clinical trial, which will be discussed next.

Figure 6.6 presents a complete list of experimental studies. These include community and clinical trials (often called medical trials). Prevention and treatment intervention trials, which are types of clinical trials, are commonly used in experimental study designs.

Clinical Trials

Clinical trials can be defined as experimental studies that attempt to determine both the efficacy and efficiency of a therapeutic agent such as a drug or a procedure. The treatment is allocated by the investigator, giving clinical trials their experimental nature. *Efficacy* measures whether the treatment improves the health of individuals who receive it. *Efficiency* measures the resources consumed by the treatment.

Clinical trials are the most common experimental study. In general, there are several types of clinical trials: therapeutic, prevention, screening, diagnostic, and quality-of-life trials. *Treatment trials* evaluate new types of treatments, which may include medications, surgery, or combinations. *Prevention trials* test new prevention methods for avoiding the risk of getting a disease. *Screening trials* (that is, early detection trials) look for better ways to identify early stages of a disease. *Diagnostic trials* search for better tests or procedures for diagnosing a particular disease or condition. *Quality-of-life trials* evaluate methods to improve the quality of life of patients who have chronic diseases.

Clinical trials have two objectives: (1) to understand whether receiving the new treatment or prevention results in a better clinical outcome than not receiving the new treatment, and (2) to determine whether a new treatment has any harmful side effects. Clinical trials must avoid bias. Because the trials aim to identify some difference in the health outcome between the treatment and control groups, any difference in this outcome should be due to the effect of the new treatment and not to any other factors. Bias is the difference observed that is due to some factor other than the new treatment.

One method to overcome bias is the use of masking. *Masking*, also known as blinding, is used to eliminate bias that may originate from any of the people involved in the clinical trials: the subject and investigator (observer). *Single-blind clinical trials* are those in which subjects do not know which group they are in, and they do not know whether they are receiving the new treatment. *Double-blind clinical trials* are those in which neither the subject nor the investigators know to which group the subject has been assigned until the conclusion of the study.

Another method to eliminate bias is to use control groups. Clinical trials can be divided into two general types, uncontrolled and controlled trials. *Uncontrolled trials* have no comparison (control) group that can be used to evaluate the new treatment. Treatments are tested on a number of subjects, and results are monitored. Results of these trials cannot be generalized to the overall population. This characteristic results in limited usefulness of the trial results.

In *controlled trials*, the results of a new treatment are compared with those of an existing treatment or with no treatment. People who receive the new treatment are called the treatment group. People who do not receive the new treatment are called the control group. Testing a new treatment against no treatment usually involves using a placebo (in terms of pharmaceuticals, a placebo is an inactive substance that appears identical to an active medication). In controlled clinical trials, the selection of people for control groups is important, both ethically and therapeutically. When the clinical trial is attempting to determine whether a new treatment results in an improvement over an existing treatment, control groups are treated by the best existing treatment. If no accepted treatment currently exists, then control groups are untreated, and the clinical trial evaluates whether the new treatment provides a better result than doing nothing.

The most important characteristic of clinical trials is the method used to select and assign people to study groups. There are several methods of allocation that can be used, including random, nonrandom, and systematic. *Random allocation* uses chance to determine assignment to study groups. *Nonrandom allocation* assigns subjects to study groups by some process that does not use chance. *Systematic allocation* is not random but is based on some criterion that is expected not to affect the outcome of the study.

Randomization is the method of assigning individuals to study groups in a manner that all possible assignments and compositions of study groups are equally likely. In other words, each person selected for the study has an equal chance of receiving either the new treatment or the existing treatment. The reason for randomization is to ensure that the two groups, the one that receives the new treatment and the one that does not, are comparable and are similar at the beginning of the clinical trial. This way, at the end of the clinical trial any difference that is seen between the two groups will be caused by the new treatment.

Randomization prevents bias, or error, that is caused by confounding characteristics of the people in a study. For example, if clinical trial subjects are people from the same neighborhood with the same race and same age group, then they are similar at the beginning. Any difference in the health outcome at the end of the trial will be caused by the differing effect of the new treatment and not by any of the possible confounding characteristics of the people in the trial.

A popular type of clinical trial is the *randomized controlled clinical trial.* A randomized controlled clinical trial uses randomization to eliminate investigator bias by randomly assigning individuals to treatment and control groups. These trials are either single- or double-blind and usually result in the most accurate estimate of treatment effect. Randomized controlled clinical trials are the most useful for comparison because of the use of randomly allocated controls.

The design of a randomized controlled clinical trial is shown in Figure 6.7. The significant characteristic is that both study subjects and controls come from the same subpopulation of individuals who volunteer for the trial. Because of randomization, the volunteer bias should be evenly distributed among both study subjects and controls, so the effect of bias should be less problematic. If a randomized controlled clinical trial is properly done, it will provide the best evidence of whether a new treatment results in a better health outcome.

An example of systematic allocation is the use of subjects' birth date. For example, all subjects born on an even-numbered birth date are assigned to the treatment group, and all subjects born on an odd-numbered birth date are assigned to the control group. The disadvantage with this method is the possibility of bias on the part of the investigator because he or she may know the birth dates, and this could affect the assignment of subjects.

Clinical trials are designed based on study needs that originate from laboratory research. After the need has been established, a clinical trial plan called a *protocol* is developed. In practice, clinical trials are organized in phases. Phase 0 trials include the administration of single doses of a study drug to a small number of subjects (usually between ten and fifteen). The purpose of phase 0 trials is to

FIGURE 6.7: Framework for a randomized clinical trial

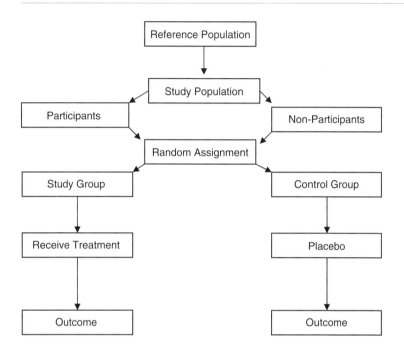

obtain preliminary information on how the body processes the drug and how the drug works in the body. Phase 0 trials are done to decide whether clinical trials should be started.

Phase I trials are the first stage of testing in humans and involve small groups (usually between twenty and eighty) of healthy people who volunteer for the study. The main purpose of phase I trials is to test the safety and tolerability, how the body processes the drug, and how the drug works in the body. Phase II trials are performed on larger groups (between eighty and three hundred). The main purpose of phase II trials is to test how well the drug works and to continue to assess the safety of the drug. Phase III trials are randomized controlled trials done on large groups (between three hundred and three thousand people). Phase III trials intend to be the defining assessment of how effective a drug works in comparison with existing drugs. Phase IV trials are known as "postmarketing surveillance trials." They are focused on safety surveillance after the drug has been approved for use. Phase IV trials are often required by regulatory authorities.

Phase 0 and Phase I drug trials use healthy volunteers. Most other clinical trials use people who have a specific disease or medical condition.

Ethical Concerns

Because of the nature of clinical trials, they are closely monitored by regulatory agencies. Clinical trials that involve a medical or therapeutic intervention on people must be first approved by an ethics committee. This local ethics committee has the authority to decide how the clinical trial will be supervised. In the United States the local ethics committee is called the *institutional review board*. These boards are usually located in the hospital or university where the clinical trial will take place.

INSTITUTIONAL REVIEW BOARDS

An institutional review board (IRB), also known as an independent ethics committee or ethical review board, is a committee that approves, monitors, and reviews biomedical and behavioral research involving humans to protect the rights and welfare of the research subjects.

The IRB reviews research projects that involve human subjects to ensure that subjects are not placed at undue risk and that human subjects give uncoerced, informed consent to their participation.

HEALTH INSURANCE PORTABILITY AND ACCOUNTABILITY ACT OF 1996 (HIPAA)

HIPAA provides federal protections for personal health information held by health care providers and insurers and gives patients rights with respect to that information. HIPAA permits the disclosure of personal health information needed for patient care and other important purposes.

Source: U.S. Department of Health and Human Services, http://www.hhs.gov/ocr/privacy/hipaa/understanding/index.html.

For a clinical trial to be considered ethical, full and informed consent from all participating human subjects must be obtained. Often the local IRB also certifies the research staff before they can conduct clinical trials. The research staff must understand the Health Insurance Portability and Accountability Act of 1996 (known as HIPAA) and good clinical practice. The staff must understand guidelines that protect the rights, safety, and well-being of all study subjects.

Bias and Validity

Clinical trials need to be accurate because their results are used to institute drug treatments and medical procedures for general use in the population. Accuracy is assessed by the measurement known as validity. *Validity* represents the truth of the clinical trial results.

VALIDITY

Validity is the extent to which a test measures a true value. The validity of a test measures its accuracy. The terms "validity" and "accuracy" are synonymous. Validity measures the truth.

Internal validity is concerned with cause-and-effect relationships. Internal validity indicates whether observed changes can be attributed to a program or intervention (that is, the cause) and not to other possible causes.

It is also important to know whether the results of a clinical trial can be used in the population. This depends on something called external validity, which indicates whether the results of a clinical trial can be generalized for use in the population. A clinical trial is externally valid if its results represent the truth for the general population.

A second consideration is whether the clinical trial is internally valid. *Internal validity* of a clinical trial refers to whether the results represent the truth for the people who participated in the trial. A clinical trial is internally valid if its results were not due to bias or chance.

Bias is actually systematic error. Systematic error occurs when the results of a clinical trial are systematically different from the truth. Bias can occur in several ways. For example, confounding bias happens when the clinical trial does not properly account for the effect of the differences among the subjects. Confounding bias can be reduced by using randomization. Measurement bias occurs when measurement methods are different between the groups in a clinical trial.

Examples of Experimental Studies

Cancer clinical trials are good examples of experimental studies. In general, there are five types of cancer clinical trials: prevention, treatment, screening and early detection, diagnosis, and quality-of-life trials. Prevention trials (referred to under "Clinical Trials") review the safety and effectiveness of risk reduction methods. Treatment trials, also referred to as therapeutic trials, evaluate the safety and effectiveness of new treatments, including drugs. Screening trials evaluate the effectiveness of new or improved ways to detect cancer in its earliest stages in people without cancer symptoms. Diagnostic trials attempt to develop better methods for identifying the types and phases of cancer, which helps in treatment and management of health care services. Quality-of-life trials (also referred to earlier) evaluate interventions that have been designed to increase the quality of life for people with cancer.

The first example is a cancer clinical trial that determined whether race had an effect on survival for men treated for prostate cancer.[11] A randomized clinical trial was done in phase III. Pretreatment and post-treatment prostate-specific antigen (PSA) values were used. The results of the trial indicated that African American men had a lower survival rate. This may have been due to higher pretreatment PSA values in African Americans.

PROSTATE-SPECIFIC ANTIGEN

Prostate-specific antigen (PSA) is a protein produced by cells of the prostate gland. The PSA test measures the level of PSA in the blood and is used to detect prostate cancer.

Low levels of PSA are normally found in the blood. Prostate cancer increases the level of PSA. Other noncancerous conditions such as prostatitis (inflammation of the prostate) and benign prostatic hyperplasia (enlargement of the prostate) can increase PSA levels.

Source: National Cancer Institute, http://www.cancer.gov/cancertopics/factsheet/Detection/PSA.

A second example is of a breast cancer clinical trial.[12] This treatment trial evaluated whether a type of chemotherapy was safe and effective in older patients. People older than sixty-five years have a high prevalence rate of breast cancer, but they do not often participate in clinical trials. Because of this, many treatments for breast cancers are not used in older patients because of lack of knowledge of the safety and effectiveness. A reason for not including older patients is the concern over adverse effects of the different treatments. A randomized clinical trial was used, and the results indicated that chemotherapy is feasible for use in older patients, and any resulting toxicity problems can be easily treated.

Another example of a treatment cancer trial involved evaluating the risk of toxicity from chemotherapy in patients with breast cancer.[13] This can be a major problem in elderly patients who have decreased kidney function because of old age. The trial looked at the creatinine levels of patients as an indicator of toxicity. The results of the trial indicated that patients with high creatinine levels had an increased risk for having fever and blood toxicity.

A final example is of a quality-of-life clinical trial for lung cancer.[14] Quality-of-life measurements provide information about a person's life as it is affected by the treatment and effects of cancer. People in phase III trials were evaluated for their quality of life. This trial concluded that some chemotherapy drugs have better quality-of-life outcomes than others.

Summary

Several different epidemiological study designs are in use today. Some of these study designs can test hypotheses that there is a relationship between risk factors and a disease. The experimental study design establishes the framework for clinical trials, which evaluate new clinical interventions to treat and prevent diseases. The randomized controlled clinical trial is most commonly used today.

Observational study designs are more commonly used. Observational studies that cannot test hypotheses include cross-sectional (also called prevalence studies) and descriptive studies. The observational studies that can test cause-and-effect hypotheses are the prospective (also called cohort) study and the retrospective (also called case-control) study.

Key Terms

Bias, 114

Cases, 118

Case report, 116

Case series, 116

Chapter Exercises

Using the information provided, determine which study design is being used. Your answers should include the general study type (experimental or observational) as well as the specific study type (descriptive, cross-sectional, ecological, case series, prospective, or retrospective).

1. A researcher is interested in the cause of neonatal jaundice. To study this condition, he selects one hundred children who were diagnosed with neonatal jaundice. He also selects another one hundred children born during the same time period at the same hospital who did not have a diagnosis of neonatal jaundice. He then reviewed the obstetrical and delivery records of their mothers to determine if there were any prenatal or perinatal exposures to risk factors.

2. In 1965 one thousand men were working in an asbestos manufacturing facility. The incidence rate of lung cancer in these men up to the year 1995 was

compared with that of one thousand men who began work as telephone repairmen in 1965. Twenty of the asbestos factory workers and four of the telephone repairmen developed lung cancer during the thirty years between 1965 and 1995.

3. A group of women attending a clinic for their first prenatal visit are enrolled in a study to determine if taking erythromycin during pregnancy adversely affects birth weight. The women are randomly put into control or experimental groups.

4. A study is done to review and understand the influence of environmental risk factors for blood lead concentrations in children. Blood specimens are taken from a selected subgroup of the children who have been identified to be high risk because they live in an inner city and are poor. At the time that the blood specimens are taken, the mothers are asked about several possible environmental exposures.

5. In 1997 five hundred men who work at a local chemical manufacturing facility were examined for coronary artery disease. The men have been examined every three years to identify new cases of coronary artery disease.

Chapter Review

1. The essential difference between an experimental and an observational study is that in an experimental study, the
   a. study and control groups are selected based on their history of risk factor exposure.
   b. study is retrospective in direction.
   c. study is prospective in direction.
   d. the study and control groups are equal in size.
   e. the investigator determines who is and who is not exposed to the risk factor.

2. Which of the following is associated with a retrospective study?
   a. It is prospective in direction.
   b. It is useful for the investigation of rarely occurring diseases.
   c. It is useful for the investigation of rarely occurring risk factor exposure.
   d. It allows for direct calculation of a disease incidence rate.
   e. None of the above.

3. Randomization is used in a clinical trial to
   a. ensure that all trial subjects have an equal chance of being assigned to the experimental or control groups.
   b. distinguish the clinical trial from a prospective study.

    c. distinguish the clinical trial from a retrospective study.

    d. ensure that the experimental and control groups are selected from the same population.

4. The purpose of a double-blind study is to

    a. achieve comparability of cases and controls.

    b. avoid bias.

    c. reduce the number of subjects who are lost to follow-up.

    d. all of the above.

5. What are the advantages of prospective studies?

6. What are the disadvantages of prospective studies?

7. What are the advantages of retrospective studies?

8. What are the disadvantages of retrospective studies?

9. Study subjects included in this type of study do not show evidence of the disease under consideration when the study begins. The study subjects are classified by whether or not they have been exposed to the risk factor. The study subjects are observed forward in time to determine the number of new cases of the disease in those with and without exposure to the risk factor. This type of study is

    a. a case series.

    b. a retrospective study.

    c. a clinical trial.

    d. a prospective study.

10. This type of study identifies a group of people who have a diagnosed disease and a group of people who do not have this disease. Information is collected from medical records and other historical data about past exposure to a risk factor. This type of study is

    a. a case series.

    b. a retrospective study.

    c. a clinical trial.

    d. a prospective study.

USES OF EPIDEMIOLOGICAL STUDIES

LEARNING OBJECTIVES

On completing this chapter, you will be able to

Discuss the concept of association between causal factors and disease
Explain the use of epidemiological studies to test cause-and-effect hypotheses
Explain the method of measuring the association between causal factors and disease
Define relative risk, attributable risk, and odds ratio

Introduction

You already have read and studied hypothesis testing, experimental studies, and observational studies in previous chapters. You have read about the different types of observational studies and how they happen. These analytical studies are used to test hypotheses about causal relationships between a risk factor and

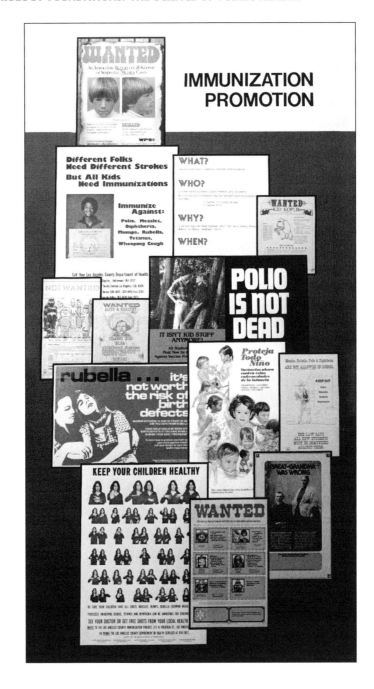

whether or not a disease develops. What hypothesis testing is trying to determine is whether a risk factor is actually one of the causes of a disease.

Observational Studies

Quantifying Cause-and-Effect Relationships

We can actually measure the impact of the relationship between risk factors and disease by determining that an association exists. You can never state directly that a risk factor causes a disease. This is because of the complex nature of the relationship between risk factors and a disease. An association can be defined as the presence of a statistical relationship that can be quantified between two or more factors and a disease. In other words, an *association* is the presence of a statistical relationship between the presence or absence of a risk factor and the presence and absence of a disease.

To explain why you can only say that an association exists between a risk factor and disease, there exists four possible situations. These are

1. the risk factor is present, and the disease is present;

2. the risk factor is absent, and the disease is absent;

3. the risk factor is present, but the disease is absent;

4. the risk factor is absent, but the disease is present.

If every time a risk factor was present the disease was present, then you could say that the risk factor causes the disease. If every time the risk factor was absent the disease was absent, then you could say the risk factor does not cause the disease. Because neither of these two situations is always the case, the most that you can say is that an association exists between a risk factor and a disease. Figure 7.1 graphically shows the relationship between a risk factor and a disease.

Risk Ratios

Risk can be thought of as the chance that a disease will develop over a defined period of time. This chance is the way that the association is quantified. The risk is a measurement of the association. Risk ratios are one of the measurements used to quantify an association. Specific risk ratios are used depending on the observational study design. For cohort studies, the risk ratio used is called the *relative risk*. The relative risk measures the association between a risk factor and

FIGURE 7.1: Relationship between risk factor and disease

1. Risk Factor is present and the Disease is present

2. Risk Factor is absent and the Disease is absent

3. Risk Factor is present but the Disease is absent

4. Risk Factor is absent but the Disease is present

a disease for cohort studies by reviewing the relationship of the incidence rate in the population.

The relative risk compares the new cases of a disease in people who have the risk factor (the situation when the risk factor is present) and people who do not have the risk factor (the situation when the risk factor is absent). In a cohort study, the incidence rate is measured in people who have been exposed to the risk factor and in people who have not been exposed. In this way, the relative risk measures the relative impact that a risk factor has on the development of a disease in people who have been and have not been exposed to the risk factor. The relative risk measures the strength of an association; the greater the chance that a risk factor causes a disease, the greater the strength of association.

The relative risk is defined as a ratio and is as follows:

$$\frac{\text{incidence rate among people who are exposed to the risk factor}}{\text{incidence rate among people who are not exposed to the risk factor}}$$

The value of the relative risk can range from 0 (no one in the exposed group develops the disease) to ∞ (all people in the exposed group will develop the disease). A relative risk *equal to 1* (which means that the ratio is *1 to 1* or that the incidence rate in the numerator is the same as the incidence rate in the denominator) tells us that the chance of the disease developing is not affected by exposure to the risk factor. A relative risk *greater than 1* (which means the incidence rate in the numerator is greater than the incidence rate in the denominator) indicates that exposure to the risk factor increases the chance of the disease developing. A relative risk *less than 1* (which means the incidence rate in the numerator is less than the incidence rate in the denominator) tells us that exposure to the risk factor decreases the chance of developing the disease.

TABLE 7.1: Relative Risk 2 × 2 Contingency Table

	New Cases of Disease	No Disease	Total
Risk factor exposure	a	b	$a + b$
No risk factor exposure	c	d	$c + d$
Total	$a + c$	$b + d$	$a + b + c + d$

$$relative\ risk = \frac{\text{incidence rate in the top row}}{\text{incidence rate in the bottom row}}$$

$$= \frac{a/(a+b)}{c/(c+d)}$$

The numerical value of the relative risk, as a ratio, may be difficult to understand. Because it is a ratio, it has no numerical units. Instead, it is expressed as the relationship between the numerator and the denominator. The value of the relative risk tells us how much the chance of developing a disease is either increased or decreased. For example, a relative risk of 5 means that the chance of a disease developing is increased five times if a person is exposed to the risk factor. A relative risk of 0.5 tells us that the chance that a disease will develop is decreased 50 percent. The relative risk is not a measure of the chance that a disease will develop but how much the chance is changed if a person is exposed to a risk factor.

Table 7.1 shows how the relative risk is calculated. The table shows a 2 × 2 contingency table that has two columns and two rows. The columns show two possible situations: the disease has developed or it has not. The left column shows the new cases, and the right column shows those in whom the disease did not develop. The rows show whether or not the people have been exposed to the risk factor. The top row contains those people who were exposed to the risk factor. The bottom row shows the people who were not exposed to the risk factor.

A 2 × 2 contingency table has four cells. The top left cell of the table (top row, left column), which is labeled a, shows the number of people who have the disease and were exposed to the risk factor. The top right cell of the table (top row, right column), which is labeled b, shows the number of people who do not have the disease but were exposed to the risk factor. The bottom left cell (bottom row, left column), which is labeled c, shows the number of people who have the disease but were not exposed to the risk factor. The bottom right cell (bottom row, right column), which is labeled d, shows the number of people who do not have the disease and were not exposed to the risk factor.

2 × 2 CONTINGENCY TABLES

2 × 2 contingency tables are used to record and analyze the relationship between two or more variables. The figures in the right-hand column and the bottom row are called marginal totals, and the figure in the bottom right-hand corner is the grand total.

TABLE 7.2: Relative Risk Calculation

	New Cases of Disease	No Disease	Total
Risk factor exposure	a 140	b 80	$a + b$ 220
No risk factor exposure	c 50	d 230	$c + d$ 280
Total	$a + b$ 190	$b + d$ 310	$a + b + c + d$ 500

$$relative\ risk = \frac{\text{incidence rate in the top row}}{\text{incidence rate in the bottom row}}$$

$$= \frac{a/(a+b)}{c/(c+d)}$$

$$= \frac{140/220}{50/280} = 3.55\ \text{to}\ 1$$

The relative risk is equal to the incidence rate in the top row divided by the incidence rate in the bottom row. That is, the relative risk is the number of people with the disease (new cases) in the top row divided by the total number of people in the top row, divided by the number of people with the disease (new cases) in the bottom row divided by the total number of people in the bottom row. The relative risk equals $(a/a + b)/(c/c + d)$.

Table 7.2 shows an example of the calculation of the relative risk. The number of people with the disease and who were influenced by the risk factor (a) equals 140, with 80 other people without the disease who were also influenced by the risk factor (b). The number of people with the disease who were not influenced by the risk factor (c) equals 50, with 230 people who did not develop the disease also not influenced by the risk factor (d). The relative risk is equal to the incidence rate in the top row divided by the incidence rate in the bottom row, or $(a/a + b)/(c/c + d)$. The relative risk is 3.55 to 1. This tells us that if a

TABLE 7.3: Relative Risk Calculation Example 1

	Lung Cancer	No Lung Cancer	Total
Smoker	a 1,500	b 8,500	a + b 10,000
Nonsmoker	c 100	d 9,900	c + d 10,000
Total	a + c 1,600	b + d 18,400	a + b + c + d 20,000

$$relative\ risk = \frac{\text{incidence rate in the top row}}{\text{incidence rate in the bottom row}}$$

$$= \frac{a/(a+b)}{c/(c+d)}$$

$$= \frac{1{,}500/10{,}000}{100/10{,}000} = \frac{0.176}{0.01} = 17.6 \text{ to } 1$$

person is affected by the risk factor, their chance of developing the disease will increase 3.55 times.

Table 7.3 presents an example of calculating the relative risk. In a population of 20,000, the effect of smoking on the development of lung cancer was studied for twenty years. The 2×2 contingency table shows the information that resulted from the study. In the population of 20,000 people, 50 percent (10,000) were smokers. Lung cancer developed in 1,500 of the smokers (a) and 100 of the nonsmokers (c). Among the smokers, 8,500 did not develop lung cancer (b). Among the nonsmokers, 9,900 did not develop lung cancer during the twenty-year study (d).

The relative risk is the ratio of the incidence rate of lung cancer among smokers to the incidence rate of lung cancer among nonsmokers. The incidence rate of lung cancer among smokers is calculated using the top row of the 2×2 table and is calculated by (a/a + b). This equals 1,500 divided by 10,000, or 0.176. The incidence rate of lung cancer among nonsmokers is calculated using the bottom row of the 2×2 table and is calculated by (c/c + d). This equals 100 divided by 9,900, or 0.01. The relative risk is calculated by (a/a + b)/(c/c + d), or 0.176 divided by 0.01, which equals 17.6 to 1. This means that people in this population who smoke have a 17.6 times greater chance of developing lung cancer than people in this population who do not smoke.

Table 7.4 presents a second example of calculating the relative risk. This example is based on a prospective study of the effect of exercise on preterm labor in a population of low-risk pregnant working women.[1] The 2×2 contingency table shows that there were 455 pregnant women in the study. The number of

TABLE 7.4: Relative Risk Calculation Example 2

	Preterm Labor	No Preterm Labor	Total
Exercise	a	b	$a + b$
	22	216	238
No exercise	c	d	$c + d$
	18	199	217
Total	$a + c$	$b + d$	$a + b + c + d$
	44	415	455

$$relative\ risk = \frac{\text{incidence rate in the top row}}{\text{incidence rate in the bottom row}}$$

$$= \frac{a/(a+b)}{c/(c+d)}$$

$$= \frac{22/238}{18/217} = \frac{0.092}{0.083} = 1.1\,to\,1$$

women who participated in regular exercise equaled 238 (these are shown in the top row). The remaining 217 did not participate in regular exercise (see bottom row). Among the women who exercised, 22 experienced preterm labor (a) and 216 did not have preterm labor (b). Among the women who did not exercise, 18 had preterm labor (c) and 199 did not experience preterm labor (d).

The incidence rate of preterm labor among women who exercised is calculated using the top row of the 2×2 table and is calculated by ($a/a + b$). This equals 22 divided by 238, or 0.092. The incidence rate of preterm labor among women who exercised is calculated using the bottom row of the 2×2 table and is calculated by ($c/c + d$). This equals 18 divided by 217, or 0.083. The relative risk is calculated by ($a/a + b$)/($c/c + d$), or 0.092 divided by 0.083, which equals 1.1 to 1. This means that the pregnant women in this population who exercise regularly have the same chance of experiencing preterm labor as do the pregnant women in this population who do not exercise.

Odds Ratio

As we did with the cohort study, one objective of the case-control study design is to determine whether an association exists between the risk factors and a disease. The incidence rate is calculated in cohort studies because of its prospective nature. Cohort studies start with no subjects having a disease and observe these people for a specified period, measuring the new cases that develop. Case-control studies have a retrospective nature; these studies compare people who

FIGURE 7.2: Odds ratio calculation

1. Risk Factor is present and the Disease is present

X

2. Risk Factor is absent and the Disease is absent

_____

3. Risk Factor is present but the Disease is absent

X

4. Risk Factor is absent but the Disease is present

have a disease with those who do not have a disease. So case-control studies do not measure new cases and do not calculate the incidence rate.

How do you measure risk in case-control studies that do not calculate the incidence rate? Because the incidence rate cannot be calculated, an alternative method is to estimate the incidence rate. In case-control studies, a risk ratio can be calculated that estimates the relative risk. This risk ratio is called the *odds ratio*.

Figure 7.2 presents an explanation of the odds ratio in terms of the relationship between the risk factor and the disease. The odds ratio is the product of situations 1 and 2 divided by the product of situations 3 and 4. This product can be thought of as follows: the odds ratio is the product of the expected situations (the risk factor and disease are present, and the risk factor and the disease are absent) divided by the product of the unexpected situations (the risk factor is present but the disease is absent, and the risk factor is absent but the disease is present).

Table 7.5 presents a 2 × 2 contingency table of a case-control study. The table resembles the one used in cohort studies, with one important difference. Instead of new cases, the table shows those who have a disease (existing cases) and those who do not have the disease (controls). The top left cell (top row, left column), labeled *a*, shows the number of people who have a disease and in the past were exposed to a risk factor. The top right cell (top row, top column), labeled *b*, shows the number of people who do not have a disease and were not exposed to the risk factor. The bottom left cell (bottom row, left column), labeled *c*, shows the number of people who have the disease but were never exposed to the risk factor. The bottom right cell (bottom row, left column), labeled *d*, shows

TABLE 7.5: Odds Ratio 2 × 2 Contingency Table

	Existing Disease (cases)	No Disease (controls)	Total
Risk factor exposure	a	b	$a + b$
No risk factor exposure	c	d	$c + d$
Total	$a + c$	$b + d$	$a + b + c + d$

$$odds\ ratio = \frac{\text{product of the cells with the expected results}}{\text{product of the cells with the unexpected results}}$$

$$= \frac{a \times d}{b \times c}$$

the number of people who do not have the disease and were never exposed to the risk factor.

As you look at the 2×2 contingency table shown in Table 7.5, see what the columns and rows are presenting. The left column shows people who have a disease (cases), and the right column shows people who do not have a disease (controls). As you think about risk factors and disease, it makes sense to expect that those people who have been exposed to a risk factor should have the disease. These people are presented in the top left cell labeled a. If you continue this line of thinking, it makes sense to expect that people who have never been exposed to a risk factor should not have the disease. These people are presented in the bottom right cell labeled d. The cells labeled b and c (the top right and bottom left cells) present situations that you would not expect. The top right cell, labeled b, shows the number of people who have been exposed to the risk factor but do not have the disease. The bottom left cell, labeled c, shows the number of people who have the disease but were never exposed to the risk factor. The odds ratio equals the product of the two expected cells (a times d), divided by the product of the two cells with the unexpected results (b times c), or

$$(a \times d)/(b \times c).$$

Table 7.6 presents the calculation of the odds ratio using the same numbers that were shown in Table 7.2. The cells with the expected situations are the number of people who have the disease and were exposed to the risk factor (cell a) equals 140, with 230 people who do not have the disease and were never exposed to the risk factor (cell d). The cells with the unexpected situations are the number of people who do not have the disease but were exposed to the risk factor (cell b) equals 80, and 50 people who have the disease and were never

TABLE 7.6: Calculation of Odds Ratio

	Cases (Existing Disease)	Controls (No Disease)	Total
Risk factor exposure	a 140	b 80	$a + b$ 220
No risk factor exposure	c 50	d 230	$c + d$ 280
Total	$a + c$ 190	$b + d$ 310	$a + b + c + d$ 500

$$\text{odds ratio} = \frac{\text{product of the cells with the expected results}}{\text{product of the cells with the unexpected results}}$$

$$= \frac{a \times d}{b \times c}$$

$$= \frac{140 \times 230}{80 \times 50} = 8.05 \text{ to } 1$$

TABLE 7.7: Odds Ratio Example 1

	Cases of Lung Cancer	Controls	Total
Smoking	a 1,000	b 4,000	$a + b$ 5,000
No smoking exposure	c 250	d 4,750	$c + d$ 5,000
Total	$a + c$ 1,250	$b + d$ 8,750	$a + b + c + d$ 10,000

$$\text{odds ratio} = \frac{\text{product of the cells with the expected results}}{\text{product of the cells with the unexpected results}}$$

$$= \frac{a \times d}{b \times c}$$

$$= \frac{1,000 \times 4,750}{250 \times 4,000} = 4.75 \text{ to } 1$$

exposed to the risk factor (cell c). The product of the expected cells ($a \times d$) divided by the product of the unexpected cells ($b \times c$), the odds ratio, equals 8.05 to 1. This means that people who have been exposed to the risk factor in the past have an 8.05 times greater chance of having the disease.

Table 7.7 shows an example of calculating the odds ratio. The 2 × 2 contingency table presents information about the relationship of smoking and lung

TABLE 7.8: Odds Ratio Example 2

	Cases of Diabetes	Controls	Total
Improper diet	a 35	b 465	a + b 500
Proper diet	c 10	d 490	c + d 500
Total	a + c 45	b + d 955	a + b + c + d 1,000

$$\text{odds ratio} = \frac{\text{product of the cells with the expected results}}{\text{product of the cells with the unexpected results}}$$

$$= \frac{a \times d}{b \times c}$$

$$= \frac{35 \times 490}{10 \times 465} = 3.68 \text{ to } 1$$

cancer in a group of 10,000 people, 5,000 smokers and 5,000 people who do not smoke. At the time the information was collected, 1,250 people had lung cancer and 8,750 people did not. Among the people with lung cancer, 1,000 were smokers. Among the people who did not have lung cancer, 4,000 were smokers. The odds ratio is the product of the expected cells ($a \times d$) divided by the product of the unexpected cells ($b \times c$). The odds ratio in this example is $(1,000 \times 4,750)/(4,000 \times 250)$, or 4.75 to 1. This means that people who have smoked in the past have a 4.75 times greater chance of having lung cancer.

Table 7.8 shows another example of calculating the odds ratio. The 2×2 contingency table presents information that was collected at a health fair on the relationship of an improper diet and diabetes in people who are at risk for diabetes developing. A total of 1,000 people who have a risk of diabetes developing were evaluated for presence of the disease. During the evaluation, 45 people were found to have diabetes. Another finding was that 500 people reported that they had an improper diet. Among those 500 people, 35 were found to have diabetes. Among the 500 people who reported having a proper diet, 10 were found to have diabetes. The odds ratio is the product of the expected cells ($a \times d$) divided by the product of the unexpected cells ($b \times c$). The odds ratio in this example is $(35 \times 490)/(10 \times 465)$, or 3.68 to 1. This means that people who are at risk for diabetes and have an improper diet have a 3.68 times greater chance of the disease developing.

Table 7.9 presents another example of calculating the odds ratio. The 2×2 contingency table shows information on the effect of smoking on the occurrence of stroke. A population of 7,872 people was studied for the effect of smoking

TABLE 7.9: Odds Ratio Example 3

	Stroke	Controls	Total
Smoking	*a* 171	*b* 3,264	*a + b* 3,435
No smoking exposure	*c* 117	*d* 4,320	*c + d* 4,437
Total	*a + c* 288	*b + d* 7,584	*a + b + c + d* 7,872

$$\text{odds ratio} = \frac{\text{product of the cells with the expected results}}{\text{product of the cells with the unexpected results}}$$

$$= \frac{a \times d}{b \times c}$$

$$= \frac{171 \times 4,320}{117 \times 3,264} = 1.93 \text{ to } 1$$

on the occurrence of a stroke. In this population, 3,435 people were smokers (top row) and 4,437 were not smokers (bottom row). Stroke had happened in 171 of the smokers (*a*) and in 117 of the people who did not smoke (*c*). The odds ratio is the product of the cells in which the expected has occurred divided by the product of the cells in which the unexpected has occurred, or (*a* × *d*)/ (*b* × *c*). The odds ratio is equal to (171 × 4,320)/(3,264 × 117), which equals 1.93 to 1. This means that people in this population who smoke have a 1.93 times greater chance of having a stroke than people in this population who do not smoke.

Attributable Risk

The impact of a risk factor can be measured by the number of people affected in a cohort study. The difference between incidence rates in those who have and have not been exposed to a risk factor is known as the *attributable risk*. The attributable risk measures the absolute difference in the incidence rates and can be calculated as

incidence rate of the people exposed to the risk factor *minus* the incidence rate of the people who were not exposed to the risk factors.

The attributable risk measures the amount of risk in the population that can be linked to a specific risk factor. It measures the increase in the number of new cases of a disease that develop because of being exposed to a risk factor. So the

TABLE 7.10: Attributable Risk Table

	New Case of Disease	No Disease	Total
Risk factor exposure	a	b	a + b
No risk factor exposure	c	d	c + d
Total	a + c	b + d	a + b + c + d

attributable risk = incidence rate in the top row *minus* the incidence rate in the bottom row

$$= (a/a+b)-(c/c+d)$$

TABLE 7.11: Attributable Risk Calculation

	New Case of Disease	No Disease	Total
Risk factor exposure	a	b	a + b
	140	80	220
No risk factor exposure	c	d	c + d
	50	230	280
Total	a + c	b + d	a + b + c + d
	190	310	500

attributable risk = incidence rate in the top row *minus* incidence rate in the bottom row

$$= (a/a+b)-(c/c+d)$$
$$= (140/220)-(50/280)$$
$$= 46 \text{ new cases per 100 people in the population}$$

attributable risk measures how a risk factor affects a population in the number of people with a disease that can be linked to their exposure to a risk factor.

Table 7.10 presents the 2×2 contingency table for the method to calculate the attributable risk. As presented previously, the incidence rate in the top row of the table is the top left cell, labeled a, divided by the total in the top row, or $a/(a + b)$. The incidence rate in the bottom row is the bottom left cell, labeled c, divided by the total in the bottom row, or $c/(c + d)$. The attributable risk is the difference between these incidence rates or $a/(a + b) - c/(c + d)$.

Table 7.11 presents the calculation of the attributable risk, using the same numbers presented Table 7.6. The incidence rate in the top row of the 2×2 contingency table is 140 divided by 220. The incidence rate in the bottom row is 50 divided by 280. The attributable risk is the incidence rate in the top row minus the incidence rate in the bottom row, or 46 new cases per 100 people

TABLE 7.12: Attributable Risk Calculation Example 1

	New Cases of Liver Dysfunction	No Liver Dysfunction	Total
Drink alcohol	a 120	b 4,880	$a + b$ 5,000
Do not drink alcohol	c 100	d 4,900	$c + d$ 5,000
Total	$a + c$ 220	$b + d$ 9,780	$a + b + c + d$ 10,000

attributable risk = incidence rate in the top row *minus* incidence rate in the bottom row

$$= (a/a+b) - (c/c+d)$$
$$= (120/5,000) - (100/5,000)$$
$$= 40 \text{ new cases per } 10,000 \text{ people in the population}$$

in the population. This indicates that 46 people per 10,000 in the population have the disease because they have been exposed to the risk factor.

An example of calculating the attributable risk is shown in Table 7.12. The 2×2 table shows information about alcohol use and liver dysfunction. The left column shows the total number of people with liver dysfunction (220), and the right column shows the total number people who do not have liver dysfunction (9,780). The top row presents the total number of people who drink alcohol (5,000), and the bottom row shows the total number of people who do not drink alcohol (5,000). The incidence rate of liver dysfunction among those people who drink alcohol is calculated using the top row. The incidence rate in the top row is 120 divided by 5,000, or 240 cases of liver dysfunction per 10,000 people in the population ($120/5,000 = 0.24 \times 10,000 = 240$ per 10,000). The incidence rate of liver dysfunction among people who did not drink alcohol is calculated using the numbers in the bottom row. The incidence rate in the bottom row is 100 divided by 4,990, or 200 cases of liver dysfunction per 10,000 people in the population ($100/5,000 = 0.20 \times 10,000 = 200$ per 10,000). The attributable risk is the incidence rate among people who drink alcohol *minus* the incidence rate among those people who do not drink alcohol. The attributable risk is calculated as follows: 240 cases of liver dysfunction per 10,000 people in the population *minus* 200 cases of liver dysfunction per 10,000 people in the population, which equals 40 cases of liver dysfunction per 10,000 people in the population ($240 - 200 = 40$). So the attributable risk is telling us that 40 cases of liver dysfunction (or 40 people with liver dysfunction) per 10,000 people in the population can be attributed to drinking alcohol.

Experimental Studies

Clinical Trial Results and Efficacy

A general objective of clinical trials is to determine whether a treatment results in a better clinical outcome than not receiving the treatment. Two goals of most clinical trials are to understand the efficacy and the safety of a drug or procedure. *Efficacy* is defined as the capacity to produce a desired effect (*American Heritage Dictionary of the English Language*, 4th edition, 2000). Another way to think of efficacy is as the extent to which some intervention (a new medication or medical procedure) produces some benefit to people during its use under ideal conditions. The question is, does a drug or procedure work? Sometimes the concept of effectiveness is confused with efficacy. Effectiveness is concerned with whether the drug or procedure works under ordinary day-to-day conditions. Effectiveness is concerned with whether to use a drug or medical procedure and whether people are helped by its use. Many times a drug or procedure is ineffective despite the fact that it is efficacious. This ineffectiveness may be caused by people's lack of acceptance of the drug or procedure, and it is not due to its not working under ideal conditions. Another cause of ineffectiveness is lack of compliance. People may not follow instructions or medical advice, which results in an ineffective drug or procedure. Effectiveness is usually measured using cohort and case-control studies.

Most clinical trials use objective measures to test the efficacy. These may include assessment of health outcomes that include a decrease in the number of hospitalizations, physician office visits, and deaths. In other words, clinical trials are usually focused on evidence of reduced morbidity and mortality. Other measures include the disappearance of clinical signs and symptoms or the decrease in a disease's effect on people. Often more general outcomes are used, such as improved health-related quality of life, which is measured by using questionnaires and surveys.

Safety

Safety is a major concern for clinical trials. Every day you hear or read about a drug that has allegedly caused harmful effects after a person begins to use it. The important point to remember is that medications can produce possible outcomes as well as risks of having adverse reactions.

Safety evaluation can include physical examinations, measurement of vital signs (blood pressure, pulse, and so forth), and laboratory test results. Specialized testing (electrocardiograms, radiological, and the like) can also be used to measure safety. Typical side effects that are seen include diarrhea and other gastrointestinal problems, shortness of breath, dizziness, muscular weakness, heart attack, stroke, and death.

Safety issues in clinical trials also involve when and how long side effects happen. Clinical trials provide information about how long it takes after beginning use of the drug or procedure for the side effects to begin. It is helpful to know which subgroups of the population are at highest risk for a harmful side effect. Another question that can be answered is about what dose of the drug caused the side effect and how long did the side effect persist after each dose. Is there a cumulative effect of the dosage on the side effect? And perhaps most important, how long did the side effect persist after the drug use was discontinued?[2]

The safety evaluation of a drug or procedure is constant and never ending as long as it is in use. In fact, side effects are often identified after the clinical trial has ended and the drug or procedure is in public use. This is seen typically with drug interactions in a large population.[3]

Summary

Epidemiological study designs are used to test hypotheses that there are cause-and-effect relationships between risk factors and a disease. The testing methods include calculating risk ratios and proportions analysis. The risk ratios quantify the relationship between risk factors and a disease. These risk ratios indicate the strength of the association between risk factors and a disease.

Risk ratios compare the incidence rates in people who have been exposed to a risk factor with those in people who have not been exposed. Prospective studies calculate the relative risk, which is a direct measure of the strength of association because the incidence rates are determined. Retrospective studies cannot determine incidence rates, but the relative risk is estimated by the odds ratio. The odds ratio is a good estimation of the relative risk in large populations.

The aim of clinical trials is to determine whether a new medical intervention is better than an existing intervention or than doing nothing. Clinical trials are used to measure the efficacy and safety of medical interventions, both treatment and preventive. Safety is an important concern both during the clinical trials and in use in large populations.

Key Terms

Attributable risk, 137

Cases, 140

Controls, 145

Efficacy, 152

Existing cases, 145

Expected situations, 145

Odds ratio, 137

Relative risk, 137

Unexpected situations, 145

Chapter Exercises

An epidemiological study investigating the association between long-term alcohol use and new cases of lung cancer collected the information presented in Table 7.13.

1. a. What is the incidence rate of lung cancer for people who use alcohol?
   b. What is the incidence rate of lung cancer for people who do not use alcohol?
   c. Calculate the relative risk of developing lung cancer in this population, given alcohol use. Show your work.

   Use the following information to answer Exercises 2 and 3: It is known that smoking is also a risk factor for lung cancer. Smoking may be a confounding factor. To eliminate the possible confounding effect of smoking on the risk of lung cancer for people who use alcohol, Table 7.14 presents the information stratified by smoking status (smokers or nonsmokers).

2. What is the relative risk of developing lung cancer among nonsmokers in this study population? Show your work.

TABLE 7.13: Lung Cancer and Alcohol Use

Use of Alcohol	Yes	No	Total
Yes	60	940	1,000
No	40	960	1,000
Total	100	1,900	2,000

TABLE 7.14: Smoking Status Stratification for Lung Cancer

Use of Alcohol	Yes	No	Total
Nonsmokers			
Yes	4	369	400
No	6	594	600
Total	10	990	1,000
Smokers			
Yes	56	544	600
No	34	366	400
Total	90	910	1,000

3. What is the relative risk of developing lung cancer among smokers in this study population? Show your work.

Chapter Review

1. The death rate per 100,000 people in the population for lung cancer is 71 in people who smoke and 7 in people who do not smoke. What is the relative risk of dying of lung cancer in smokers compared with nonsmokers?
2. The death rate per 100,000 people in the population for lung cancer is 71 in people who smoke and 7 in people who do not smoke. What is the attributable risk of dying of lung cancer in smokers compared with nonsmokers?
3. An odds ratio from a retrospective study estimates the
    a. ratio of the risk of disease in the group exposed to the risk factor with the risk of disease in the group who was not exposed to the risk factor.
    b. risk of disease in the group exposed to the risk factor.
    c. attributable risk.
    d. none of the above.
4. In a prospective study, 2,000 were studied for twenty years. During this period, 100 people developed lung cancer and of those, 90 were smokers. Of the 1,900 people who did not develop lung cancer, 710 were nonsmokers. What is the relative risk of lung cancer for smokers compared with nonsmokers?
    a. 15.4
    b. 4.0
    c. 5.06
    d. 24.8
    e. none of the above

5. In a retrospective study of 500 people, 150 where shown to have coronary artery disease, and 105 of those had a history of smoking. Of those who did not have coronary artery disease, 30 were smokers. The odds ratio of coronary artery disease for smokers compared with nonsmokers is
   a. 15.4
   b. 4.0
   c. 5.06
   d. 24.8
   e. none of the above

6. In a prospective study of a disease, the study group originally selected consisted of
   a. people who have the disease.
   b. people without the disease.
   c. people with a family history of the disease.
   d. none of the above.

7. To investigate the association between smoking and stroke, hospital records were examined for 100 people who had a stroke and 100 people who did not. The hospital records were reviewed to determine who were smokers. This is an example of a
   a. prospective study.
   b. case series.
   c. retrospective study.
   d. clinical trial.
   e. case report.

8. A researcher interested in whether a new high blood pressure drug works better than the standard medication gave 50 percent of patients the new drug and 50 percent the standard medication. This is an example of a
   a. prospective study.
   b. case series.
   c. retrospective study.
   d. clinical trial.
   e. case report.

9. A study identified 1,000 people who smoked and 1,000 people who were nonsmokers. These 2,000 people were observed for ten years to determine the number of new cases of heart disease. This is an example of a
   a. prospective study.
   b. case series.
   c. retrospective study.
   d. clinical trial.
   e. case report.

10. A physician published the details of an unusual case of rash in an adult that is typically only seen in children. This is an example of a
    a. prospective study.
    b. case series.
    c. retrospective study.
    d. clinical trial.
    e. case report.

EPIDEMICS

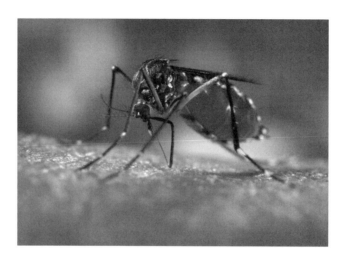

LEARNING OBJECTIVES

On completing this chapter, you will be able to

Define epidemic
Describe methods of infectious disease transmission
Describe response to epidemics
Discuss surveillance and its dependence on epidemiology
Describe reportable disease surveillance

Definition

An *epidemic*, also known as an *outbreak*, is the unexpected increase in the number of new cases of a disease at a given place or among a specific group of people during a particular time. Usually the cases have a common cause or are related in some way. Epidemics happen in large populations, and outbreaks occur in smaller populations, such as those who attend a school. However, the terms epidemic and outbreak can be used interchangeably. The major concern of epidemics is person-to-person spread of the disease. The specific number of new cases that are required to declare a situation an epidemic depends on the disease. For example, if one case of yellow fever was observed in the United States, this would be an epidemic because a case of yellow fever has not been seen since 1924, and this case was imported from another country.[1] Some diseases have many new cases a year, but this does not signify an epidemic. An example is pneumonia during the winter months.

As was mentioned in an earlier chapter, epidemics were the reason that epidemiology as a science was started. The historical purpose of epidemiology is the investigation of epidemics and the causal factors. The impact of epidemics and infectious diseases has gradually declined since the early 1900s, but infectious disease epidemics are still important, and they are associated with a majority of acute diseases.

The impact of epidemics can be measured by two epidemiological numbers, the attack rate and the secondary attack rate. The *attack rate* is the total number of new cases of a disease that occur during the epidemic period divided by the total number of people in that population during the epidemic. The attack rate is the incidence rate during the epidemic and is defined as the number of new cases of a disease during a specified period (the epidemic period) versus the total number of susceptible persons in a population during a specified period (the epidemic period).

The *secondary attack rate* is defined as the number of new cases of a disease that develop after the epidemic has ended, yet are related to the epidemic. These new cases result from exposure to infectious disease agents during the epidemic period. That is, the new cases develop during a period after the original number of cases return to the expected amount, but without exposure during the epidemic, they would not have developed.

The study of epidemics is focused on the characteristics and actions of infectious disease agents. Intrinsic characteristics allow us to differentiate between infectious disease agents and help to explain the effects on the infection process. If intrinsic characteristics are known or can be identified, then understanding an infectious agent's process (for example, mode of transmission) is straightforward.

Characteristics of the infectious disease agents that are due to the interaction with a host are important. A *host* is a person from whom the infectious disease agent obtains its nutrition to grow or shelter. These characteristics include pathogenicity, infectivity, virulence, and immunogenicity. These characteristics are dependent on several factors involving the environment and the individual host. *Pathogenicity* is the ability of the infectious disease agent to cause detectable disease and is measured by determining the ratio of the number of individuals with clinical disease to the total number of individuals who are infected by the agent. This ratio measures the number of infected individuals who actually become sick due to the presence of the infectious agent and is calculated by using the following percentage:

$$\frac{\text{total number of people with clinical disease}}{\text{total number of infected people}} \times 100$$

Infectivity is the ability of an infectious disease agent to invade and multiply in a host, which results in the infection. *Virulence* measures the severity of the infection and can be defined as the proportion of cases of clinical disease that result in severe disease or death. The case-fatality rate is typically used to measure the virulence of an infectious agent. The *case-fatality rate* is defined as follows:

$$\frac{\text{total number of deaths from an infectious disease}}{\text{total number of people infected}}$$

Immunogenicity is defined as the ability of an infection to produce specific immunity. Immunogenicity is affected by host factors (age, nutrition, and so on) as well as dose and virulence of the infection.

Transmission

Transmission is the process of passing an infectious disease from one infected person to a group of people who are not infected. There are two types of transmission mechanisms for infectious disease agents. The first type is called *direct transmission,* which is the immediate transfer of an infectious agent from one host to another person through a portal of entry. Direct transmission activities include direct physical contact, kissing, and sexual intercourse. Direct contact can also occur by droplet contact or by coughing or sneezing on another person.

Diseases that can be transmitted by direct contact (including kissing) are called *contagious diseases*. They include athlete's foot, impetigo, syphilis, cytomegalovirus infections, herpes simplex infections, mononucleosis, and warts. Diseases that can be spread by coughing or sneezing include bacterial meningitis, chickenpox, common cold, influenza, mumps, strep throat, tuberculosis, measles, rubella, and whooping cough. Diseases that can be spread by sexual intercourse include HIVS/AIDS, chlamydia, genital warts, gonorrhea, hepatitis B, and syphilis.

SEXUALLY TRANSMITTED DISEASES

Chlamydia is a common STD caused by the bacterium *Chlamydia trachomatis*. Chlamydia can damage a woman's reproductive organs.

Genital herpes is an STD caused by the herpes simplex viruses type 1 (HSV-1) and type 2 (HSV-2). Symptoms are often not seen, but when they occur, they appear as blisters on or around the genitals or rectum. The blisters break, leaving tender ulcers (sores) that may take two to four weeks to heal the first time they occur.

Trichomoniasis is an STD caused by a single-celled protozoan parasite, *Trichomonas vaginalis*. The vagina is the most common site of infection in women and the urethra in men.

Source: Centers for Disease Control and Prevention, http://www.cdc.gov/std/general.

The second type of transmission is called *indirect transmission*. Indirect contact, which occurs from touching contaminated soil or surfaces, is an example of indirect transmission. Other ways of indirect transmission include vehicle-borne, vector-borne, and airborne transmission. *Vehicle-borne transmission* occurs through exposure to contaminated food and water. *Vector-borne transmission* occurs when the infectious disease agent is transmitted by an organism to a susceptible host. Usually vector-borne transmission occurs through insects (mosquitoes) or animals. The vector's role in the infection process may be to transport the infectious disease agent, but the vector may also provide shelter and a place for growth.

Airborne transmission

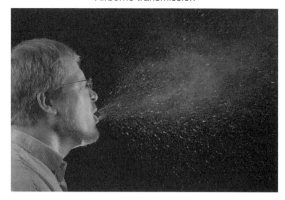

Vector-borne transmission

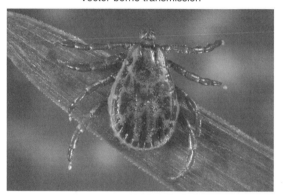

Vehicle-borne transmission

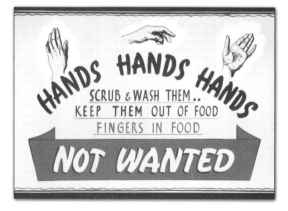

Infectious disease agents can be transmitted through the air in the form of dust and drop nuclei. Dust results from the resuspension of particles from household surfaces and soil. Droplet nuclei are tiny particles that have been formed by evaporation of sneezes, evaporation of coughed droplets, and aerosolization of infectious material.

Diseases that are spread through indirect transmission are those that occur by contact with contaminated food and water, which may result from poor hygiene or inadequate sanitary conditions. These diseases include cholera, hepatitis A, polio, rotavirus infection, and salmonellosis.

Epidemics can be divided into two types depending on their duration. *Common-source epidemics* are those caused by exposure of a group of people to the same infectious disease agent at the same point in time. Common-source epidemics are also known as a *point-source epidemic* because exposure to the infectious disease agent happens at one point in time. An example of a common-source epidemic is a food-borne outbreak such as *Salmonella enteritidis* infections associated with eggs. Figure 8.1 presents an epidemic curve for a common-source outbreak and shows that most cases occur in a short window of time.

FIGURE 8.1: Common-source epidemic

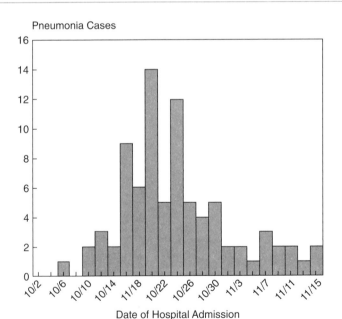

Source: Centers for Disease Control and Prevention

FIGURE 8.2: Propagated epidemic: Estimated number of AIDS cases in adults and adolescents, United States, 1985 to 2006

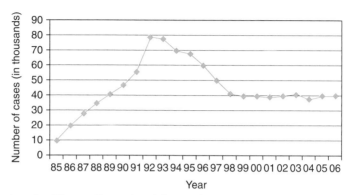

Source: Centers for Disease Control and Prevention.

The second type of epidemic is called a *propagated epidemic*. Propagated epidemics occur when susceptible people are exposed to an infectious disease agent not at the same time but over a period of time. Propagated epidemics result from the transmission, either directly or indirectly, of an infectious disease agent from one susceptible host to another person. Propagated epidemics can take place over a long time, even decades. AIDS is a propagated epidemic. Figure 8.2 presents a graphic description of a propagated epidemic.

Response to Epidemics

Investigation of an Epidemic

When an epidemic is suspected, there are ten steps that must be done to investigate it. This suspicion is usually caused by a report of an epidemic at a specific place and point in time. The ten steps to epidemic investigation are

1. Prepare to go to the place where the suspected epidemic has been reported.

2. Verify that an epidemic truly is happening.

3. Verify that the cases of disease are actually the expected disease.

4. Establish and identify the number of cases.

5. Evaluate the information obtained from the investigation as to person, place, and time.

6. Formulate hypotheses from the information.

7. Evaluate and test hypotheses.

8. If needed, refine the hypotheses and obtain additional information.

9. Begin control and prevention measures.

10. Distribute the investigation's results to the public.

In step 1, preparations must be made before going to the place where the suspected epidemic is occurring. This preparation has several parts. Information about the disease must be obtained (time duration of the disease, characteristics of the infectious disease agent, and the like). If travel is required, then the proper arrangements must be made, including how many people should be on the investigation team. The team must contact local authorities to determine their role in the investigation after they arrive at the site of the suspected epidemic.

During step 2, it must be decided if an epidemic is truly happening. To do this, you must first understand the expected number of cases of the disease for the area and at the time of year. If the number of cases seen in the area exceeds what is expected, then an epidemic is occurring. This can be determined by comparing the number of cases observed with the number of cases occurring over the past few weeks, months, or past year at the same time. This information is available from many sources, including notifiable disease surveillance that is usually done by local and state health departments. In addition, information is often obtained from hospital discharge records, death certificates, and cancer registries. If local information is not available, the team must make estimates based on data from other states in the region or national information. Other information is needed to declare that an epidemic is occurring, such as the severity of the disease and the possibility for spread of the epidemic.

In step 3, the specific disease diagnosis must be verified to be sure that the disease that is thought to be occurring is the correct one. The purpose of verification is to ensure that the problem has been properly diagnosed and that the increase in cases is not due to a diagnostic laboratory error. Verification requires the review of clinical findings (signs and symptoms) and laboratory results. Often specialized laboratory testing may be needed to be sure of the correct diagnosis. Affected people must be visited and interviewed about their exposures in the recent past. These interviews often provide information that can be used to generate hypotheses about the cause, the infectious agent, and the spread of the disease epidemic.

Step 4 involves the definition and identification of cases of the disease. In this step, a case definition is established. A *case definition* is a set of criteria used by public health agencies in the monitoring and surveillance of diseases. Case definitions are established in the CDC. A case definition has the following parts: clinical information about the disease, characteristics about the people who are affected by the disease, information about where the cases are located, and when the outbreak is occurring. For example, the case definition for AIDS is "all human immunodeficiency virus (HIV)-infected adolescents and adults aged greater than or equal to 13 years who have either (a) less than 200 CD4-positive T lymphocytes/μL [microliter]; (b) a CD4-positive T-lymphocyte percentage of total lymphocytes of less than 14%; or (c) any of the following three clinical conditions: pulmonary tuberculosis, recurrent pneumonia, or invasive cervical cancer."[2]

The case definition may be more specific in time and place for an outbreak in a small population. For example, the time element in the case definition may be less than two weeks and restricted to people who ate at a specific restaurant if a food-related outbreak is suspected. The case definition must be broad so that all the actual cases related to the outbreak are identified. All true cases must have laboratory confirmation of the effect of the disease, as seen above in the case definition for AIDS T-lymphocyte confirmation. Some patients may not have many clinical signs or symptoms, so laboratory confirmation is needed.

After the case definition has been established, cases must be identified and counted. The difficulty is that the first few cases of an epidemic are not easily identified because of their small number compared with all the cases. Also, because it takes some time to realize that an epidemic is happening, the investigation usually starts long after the epidemic has begun. The cases are identified through several sources, including hospitals, physicians' offices, and health department clinics. The investigation team must communicate the case definition to these sources and alert them that an epidemic is occurring. Information about cases must be gathered by the investigation team from all possible sources. Sometimes the health departments alert the public directly, especially when outbreaks are started by contaminated food or milk.

It is during this step that the attack rate is calculated based on the number of identified cases. The attack rate, which is the incidence rate during the epidemic period, is useful to understand the impact of the epidemic in the number of people affected and the rate at which new cases are developing.

When identifying cases, the names and addresses of cases must be obtained so a geographical map can be created. The age, sex, race, and occupation of

FIGURE 8.3: Legionnaires' disease outbreak

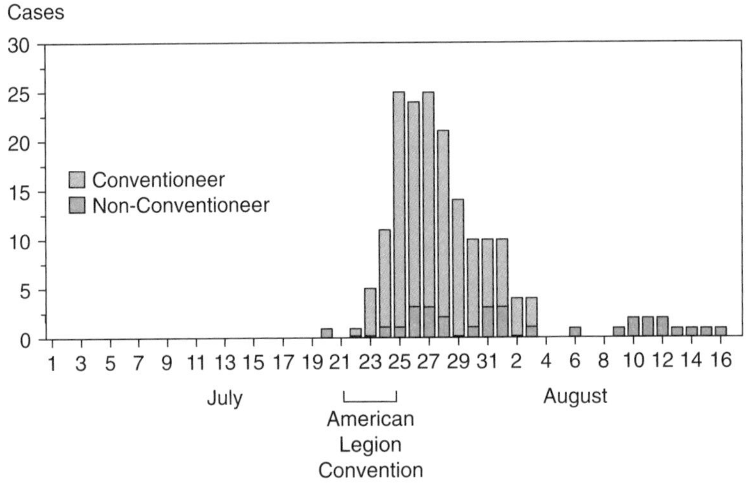

Source: Centers for Disease Control and Prevention.

patients is needed so that an idea of who is at risk can be established. Clinical information must be recorded to verify the case definition. Finally, information about the risk factors allow for the design of the investigation of the disease.

Step 5 includes the description of the epidemic, paying close attention to the person (who is affected), place (where the epidemic is occurring), and time (when it started and how long the epidemic has been happening). In this step, the epidemic curve is drawn to give a graphic view of its time trend. The epidemic curve is drawn by plotting the cases according to when they were identified. The number of cases is plotted on the y-axis, and the time is on the x-axis. Figure 8.3 shows an epidemic curve for a suspected Legionnaires' disease outbreak in 1989. In this outbreak, more than fifty cases of acute pneumonia were identified among the people of a small town in the southern United States. Most of the cases occurred during a three-week period in October.[3]

The epidemic curve provides a great deal of information. It tells you at what point the epidemic is progressing and what is its future course. It also can tell you the probable incubation period of the infectious disease agent. You can estimate from the epidemic curve what type of epidemic is occurring, point source or propagated. A point-source epidemic curve will have a steep slope and a single peak because the cases are exposed to the same source over a short period. Figure 8.3 is an example of a point-source epidemic. A propagated-epidemic curve will not have a steep slope or a single peak because there is a long period of exposure to the infectious disease agent. In addition, propagated epidemics are characterized by person-to-person spread of the disease, which results in a long, and possibly more than one, peak of the epidemic curve.

Step 6 uses the descriptive information to formulate hypotheses based on the knowledge of the disease. Hypotheses are generated to evaluate the source of the infectious disease agent, the specific method of transmission, and how people were exposed to the infectious disease. The epidemic curve should be used to help generate hypotheses.

In step 7, the hypotheses are evaluated by using analytical epidemiological methods. Prospective or retrospective study designs may be used. *Prospective studies* compare people who have been exposed to the infectious disease agent with people who have not been exposed. Prospective studies are used in epidemics that occur in small populations because it is easier to study all the people and to calculate accurate attack rates in the exposed and not-exposed groups. *Retrospective studies* compare infected people (cases) with people who do not have the disease (controls). Controls must be carefully chosen because they must be similar to cases, except that they do not have the disease. Controls and cases must be from the same population, and hypotheses must be tested using statistical methods.

Sometimes the hypotheses cannot be confirmed using analytical epidemiological studies. When this happens, step 8 is needed in which the original hypotheses are modified and additional information is obtained. Patients should be interviewed, and the new information must be used to generate new or revised hypotheses. These new hypotheses then must be evaluated following the method outlined above.

During step 9, control and prevention measures and interventions are implemented. Step 9 may begin as early in the investigation as the source of the epidemic is identified. Control and prevention measures target ways in which the epidemic can be quickly ended. Measures may be centered on eliminating the source of the infection. An example is to control a food-borne epidemic by destroying all contaminated food. Control and prevention measures may also focus on reducing the susceptibility of the population. This can be done by immunization of the population.

The last step, step 10, is to communicate the findings of the investigation team. The communication typically happens in two ways: media briefing by local health department officials and a written report. The communications should include information about what the investigation team did and the results of their investigation. The communications should mention recommendations for control and preventive measures.

Surveillance

Surveillance is the continuous evaluation of the health and disease status of populations and the identification of the occurrence of diseases. Surveillance is also concerned with the continual observation of conditions that increase the risk of disease transmission. Surveillance programs are characterized by the following: systematic collection, aggregation and formatting, analysis, and dissemination of data. Surveillance programs collect information, and then the data are aggregated and formatted into meaningful arrangements for interpretation and detailed analysis. The purpose of the data analysis is to describe trends and to test hypotheses about the disease occurrence.

Historically surveillance programs have been directed at communicable and infectious diseases. Today this still is the case, but some programs are being modified to include nosocomial infection (diseases contracted while under medical care) surveillance in hospitals, postmarketing pharmaceutical drug surveillance, and the different categories of unintentional injuries.

Disease surveillance is classified according to the target of the surveillance. The two types of surveillance are general population or *sentinel surveillance*. An entire community is the target of general population surveillance. General population surveillance is expensive, requires a large workforce, and often results in limited information. This type of surveillance is useful when it is repeated (for example, the National Household Interview Survey, which is done annually by the National Center for Health Statistics).

Sentinel surveillance targets selected sites or subpopulations. Information collected in sentinel surveillance is used to provide an assessment of the effect of interventions in a population. The results of sentinel surveillance can only be used for the specific study sites and cannot be used to make recommendations for the overall population.

Surveillance programs can be classified based on the manner in which the programs are conducted. These two types of surveillance programs are active and passive. *Active surveillance* programs seek out cases of disease by periodic contact with health care providers. They are expensive and require a great deal of time, but they provide complete data on the occurrence of diseases. *Passive surveillance* programs obtain information from laboratories or health care providers and do not actively seek out disease data. Passive surveillance programs rarely provide complete information, even over a long period. Unfortunately, this is the usual manner in which disease surveillance is carried out.

What criteria are used to decide which diseases should be placed under surveillance? The most important criterion is if prevention strategies are available for the disease. If they are not, then knowledge about the occurrence of the disease will not be useful for control. Another criterion is whether the diseases are work-related. Surveillance programs that target work-related diseases and injuries have resulted in work-practice changes to reduce risk, including the use of safety equipment, such as hard hats, steel-toed shoes, and lumbar supports. Work-related diseases may have national public health importance due to their severity and frequency, or they may be important to individual health care providers. Examples of these diseases are silicosis (respiratory tract disease caused by inhaling silica dust) and carpal tunnel syndrome.

Reportable Diseases

The National Notifiable Diseases Surveillance System was established in the United States by an Act of Congress in 1878. This surveillance system was started to obtain information about morbidity due to cholera, smallpox, plague, and yellow fever from other countries. The purpose of this information was to begin planning for quarantine programs to prevent new diseases from entering the United States. By 1912 the U.S. Public Health Service was established and monthly reporting, with telegraph contact, of ten additional notifiable diseases was begun. By 1929 the first annual summary of notifiable diseases listed twenty-nine diseases from nineteen states. The list, which includes AIDS, hepatitis, and botulism, has grown to sixty diseases today.

The list of nationally notifiable diseases is presented in Table 8.1. This list is revised periodically when a disease may be removed if the incidence rate decreases and if a new disease is added. Reporting of notifiable diseases to the CDC is voluntary by state; however, each state has laws governing mandatory reporting. All states must report the diseases requiring quarantine (those mandated by the World Health Organization), which are cholera, plague, and yellow fever. Table 8.2 presents the diseases that are monitored by WHO.

Examples

A good example of a recent epidemic is severe acute respiratory syndrome (SARS). SARS is a global infectious disease that has caused outbreaks since 2003. It is a viral respiratory tract infection caused by a coronavirus and was first reported in Asia in February 2003. In that year, SARS spread to North America, South America, Europe, and other parts of Asia. People in the United States

TABLE 8.1:   Nationally Notifiable Diseases, 2009

Acquired immunodeficiency syndrome (AIDS)	Poliomyelitis, paralytic and nonparalytic
Anthrax	Psittacosis
Arboviral neuroinvasive and noninvasive diseases (e.g., West Nile virus)	Q fever
	Rabies
Botulism	Rocky Mountain spotted fever
Brucellosis	Rubella
Chancroid	Salmonellosis
Chlamydia trachomatis infection	Severe acute respiratory syndrome (SARS)
Cholera	Shiga toxin-producing *Escherichia coli* (STEC)
Coccidioidomycosis	
Cryptosporidiosis	Shigellosis
Cyclosporiasis	Smallpox
Diphtheria	*Staphylococcus aureus* (VISA)
Ehrlichiosis or anaplasmosis	Streptococcal disease, invasive, group A
Giardiasis	
Gonorrhea	Streptococcal toxic-shock syndrome
Haemophilus influenzae infection	*Streptococcus pneumoniae,* drug-resistant
Hansen's disease (leprosy)	*Streptococcus pneumoniae,* non-drug-resistant, in children younger than 5 years
Hantavirus pulmonary syndrome	
Hemolytic uremic syndrome (postdiarrheal)	
	Syphilis
Hepatitis A, B, C (acute and chronic)	Congenital syphilis
HIV infection	Tetanus
Influenza-associated pediatric mortality	Toxic-shock syndrome (other than streptococcal)
Legionellosis	
Listeriosis	Trichinosis
Lyme disease	Tuberculosis
Malaria	Tularemia
Measles	Typhoid fever
Meningococcal disease	Vancomycin-intermediate
Mumps	Vancomycin-resistant *Staphylococcus aureus* (VRSA)
Novel influenza A virus infections	
Pertussis	Varicella (morbidity and deaths)
Plague	Vibriosis
	Yellow fever

Source: U.S. Department of Health and Human Services, Centers for Disease Control and Prevention, 2009.

TABLE 8.2: Diseases Under Surveillance by the World Health Organization, 2009

Targeted for eradication or elimination
Poliomyelitis
Dracunculiasis
Neonatal tetanus
Leprosy

Epidemic-prone diseases
Cholera
Bacillary dysentery
Plague
Yellow fever
Meningococcal meningitis
Viral hemorrhagic fever

Diseases that are a major public health problem
Diarrhea (children younger than 5 years)
Pneumonia (children younger than 5 years)
HIV/AIDS
Malaria
Trypanosomiasis
Tuberculosis
Onchocerciasis

Source: World Health Organization, Geneva: http://www.who.int/topics/public _health_surveillance/en.

had laboratory-confirmed exposure to SARS, but no cases were found in the United States. These people had traveled to areas of the world where SARS was actively transmitted. Between November 2002 and July 2003, a total of 8,098 probable SARS cases were reported to WHO from twenty-nine countries. There has been no known transmission of SARS since April 2004.

SARS symptoms include high temperature, headache, body aches, and overall discomfort. A small percentage of people had diarrhea. People with SARS develop a deep cough and pneumonia, and about 10 percent of SARS cases end in death. The incubation period can be as long as fourteen days.

SARS is an example of a propagated epidemic because it is transmitted by person-to-person contact. The SARS virus can be transmitted directly by respiratory droplets that result from sneezing and coughing at close proximity (up to three feet). It is also thought that the SARS virus can be transmitted indirectly by coming into contact with droplets on contaminated surfaces.

What makes SARS so dangerous is that it is an infectious disease that has an overall adverse effect on hospital and health care workers. Most SARS cases occur in people who care for or live with SARS patients or have direct contact with infectious materials. To add to this concern, there currently is no effective treatment for SARS. SARS patients are isolated until they are no longer infectious, with seriously affected patients admitted to hospitals.

Another example of an epidemic is West Nile virus infection, which was first seen in the West Nile region of Uganda in 1937. The global impact of the West Nile virus was first documented in 1957 when the virus was found to cause severe human meningoencephalitis. West Nile virus was first seen as an equine disease in Egypt and France during the 1960s. Recent human outbreaks have occurred in Algeria (1994), Romania (1996–1997), the Czech Republic (1997), the Democratic Republic of the Congo (1998), Russia (1999), the United States (1999–2003), and Israel (2000).

West Nile virus infection presents itself as a mild disease in most people and is characterized by flulike symptoms. Fever may be present, but it lasts only a few days with no apparent long-term effects. The most severe manifestation of West Nile virus is encephalitis, meningitis, or meningoencephalitis.

Table 8.3 shows West Nile virus activity in the United States during 2008; a total of 1,301 cases of West Nile virus were reported. Of those, 602 cases, or 46 percent, were reported as meningitis or encephalitis. About half of the cases (650) were reported as fever, and the remainder could not be clinically specified. This high percentage of reported cases with severe disease (meningitis or encephalitis) is caused by the fact that severe cases are almost always reported. It is expected that most West Nile virus infections are not reported because of the mild disease symptoms. In fact, it has been estimated that less than 10 percent of all cases will develop into severe disease.[4]

Summary

An epidemic, which is called an outbreak if it occurs in a small population, is an unexpected number of new cases of a disease. The effect of an epidemic is measured by the attack rate, which is the incidence rate during the epidemic time period. The secondary attack rate is used to understand the full extent of an epidemic.

Epidemics can spread by direct or indirect transmission. Epidemics continue until the number of susceptible people decreases. Diseases that can result in an epidemic are mandated by law to be reported when they are observed. These reportable diseases are constantly monitored by active and passive surveillance systems.

TABLE 8.3: West Nile Virus Cases, Selected States, 2008

	Encephalitis or Meningitis	Fever	Other	Total
Alabama	10	11	0	21
Arizona	53	34	10	97
Arkansas	8	0	0	8
California	252	131	9	392
Colorado	13	64	0	77
Connecticut	5	2	1	8
Idaho	1	26	6	33
Illinois	11	4	4	19
Kansas	6	26	0	32
Louisiana	9	27	0	36
Maryland	7	6	1	14
Michigan	11	4	2	17
Minnesota	3	18	0	21
Mississippi	32	66	1	99
Missouri	11	7	0	18
Nebraska	5	44	0	49
New York	31	13	0	44
Ohio	16	2	1	19
Oregon	3	13	0	16
South Dakota	11	28	0	39
Texas	37	23	0	60
Utah	6	17	1	25

Source: Centers for Disease Control and Prevention, Center for Vector-Borne Infectious Diseases, 2008.

Key Terms

Active surveillance, 170

Attack rate, 160

Case definition, 167

Case-fatality rate, 161

Common-source epidemics, 164

Contagious diseases, 162

Direct transmission, 161

Epidemic, 160

Host, 161

Immunogenicity, 161

Indirect transmission, 162

Infectivity, 161

Outbreak, 160

Passive surveillance, 170

Pathogenicity, 161

Point-source epidemic, 164

Propagated epidemic, 165

Prospective studies, 169

Chapter Exercises

1. Briefly describe the steps in the investigation of an outbreak.
2. Discuss the two types of infectious disease transmission.
3. List and describe the characteristics of an infectious disease agent.

Chapter Review

1. Disease surveillance is conducted to provide information
   a. for determining allocation of health resources.
   b. that leads to initiation of appropriate interventions.
   c. to be used to forecast future trends in health and disease.
   d. to evaluate the effectiveness of interventions.
   e. all of the above
2. In an attempt to identify cases of AIDS, state health department staff make weekly telephone calls to infection control officers in hospitals around the state. This type of surveillance is called
   a. active.
   b. passive.
   c. calibration.
   d. hospital.
3. Infectivity of an infectious agent is the
   a. ability of the agent to invade a host and multiply.
   b. ability of the agent to cause detectable disease.
   c. ability of the agent to produce specific immunity.
   d. all of the above.
   e. none of the above.
4. Pathogenicity of an infectious agent is the
   a. ability of the agent to invade a host and multiply.
   b. ability of the agent to cause detectable disease.
   c. ability of the agent to produce specific immunity.
   d. all of the above.
   e. none of the above.

5. Immunogenicity of an infectious agent is the
   a. ability of the agent to invade a host and multiply.
   b. ability of the agent to cause detectable disease.
   c. ability of the agent to produce specific immunity.
   d. all of the above.
   e. none of the above.
6. Common-source epidemics
   a. can be traced to one source at the same point in time.
   b. can be traced from person to person over a long time.
   c. are also called propagated epidemics.
   d. all of the above.
   e. none of the above.
7. Propagated epidemics
   a. can be traced to one source at the same point in time.
   b. can be traced from person to person over a long time.
   c. are also called point-source epidemics.
   d. all of the above.
   e. none of the above.
8. The first step in investigating an epidemic is
   a. deciding whether an epidemic is occurring.
   b. collecting information about the usual incidence rate of a disease.
   c. collecting information about the suspected infectious agents, and duration of the disease.
   d. all of the above.
9. Name the two types of surveillance and describe their uses.
10. Passive surveillance usually results in complete information about the occurrence of diseases. True or False?

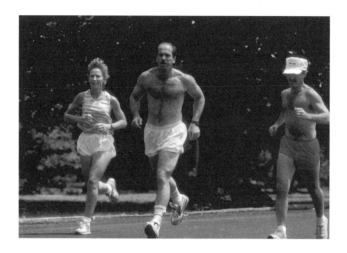

CHAPTER 9

EPIDEMIOLOGY AND SOCIETY

LEARNING OBJECTIVES

On completing this chapter, you will be able to

Define social epidemiology
Discuss what is meant by social determinants
Describe the effect of social determinants on health and disease
Describe the effect of the built environment on health and disease

Introduction

How social conditions influence health in populations has become a subject of concern over the past few decades. This concern has been caused by the need to recognize the wide spectrum of health determinants: physical, mental, and social. Epidemiology is not the only science that studies populations. Others include sociology, human biology, and population genetics.

The threat of disease in people is affected by the risk in the population and by the place where they live. Today the social aspect of everyday life is included in epidemiological investigations. The following questions must be answered: "Why does a population have high or low risk for a particular disease?" and "Why did a particular person get sick?"[1]

Social epidemiology is a relatively new branch of epidemiology that studies the influence of society on health. *Social epidemiology* is defined as "the study of the social distribution and social determinants of states of health."[2] As such, it evaluates the frequency and distribution of social conditions and their effect on health in a population.

The primary interest of social epidemiology is the study of how society influences the health and wellness of people and populations. It does this by merging traditional epidemiological concepts with economics, sociology, demography, and biology. This merger allows for the inclusion of the social experience of populations into the traditional cause-and-effect relationship. The merger allows for a better understanding of how, where, and why social inequalities affect health. A goal of social epidemiology is to explain the relationship between exposure to social conditions and its effect on health.

Society can affect a person's quality of life. People who have an available social support system have a higher rating of health-related quality of life, in both physical and mental aspects. In fact, when people with a disease were compared with people who were healthy, the sick people were found to have low health-related quality of life and less access to social support systems.[3]

It is important to understand social networks and their impact on health. A social network consists of individuals who are connected by friendship, kinship, sexual relationships, beliefs, or financially. Social networks are groups of people seen in rural communities and urban neighborhoods, including workplaces and schools.[4] Social networks have been shown to directly affect the health of people within the network. Social connections can both positively and negatively affect health, depending on the people in the network. Studies have shown that a nonbiological relationship exists between health and social networks.[5]

Social Determinants

Socioeconomic Position

We know that socioeconomic position in the population affects health. Socioeconomic position combines many characteristics, including income and educational level. In general, socioeconomic position can be looked at as a broad-based indicator of the effect on health. Knowledge of a person's socioeconomic position in the population can be used to predict lifestyle habits and activities as well as health status.

Several interesting findings have resulted from the study of socioeconomic position. For example, men and women with less than a high school education have a higher incidence of lung cancer than others who attended college. Overall, socioeconomic position showed a reverse relationship with the incidence of lung cancer and the stage of cancer at the time of diagnosis. As socioeconomic position declined, the lung cancer incidence rate and stage of cancer at diagnosis increased.[6]

Socioeconomic position has been suggested as a cause of an increased risk for coronary heart disease. Heart attacks and other coronary events were seen more frequently in people in lower socioeconomic positions in the population. This was due in part to poor lifestyle habits, which included smoking and poor nutrition.[7] For example, smoking prevalence is more than three times higher in people who have not completed high school than in high school graduates.[8]

Income

The income of people has an effect on their health. This can be explained in part by the idea that higher income allows people to buy needed health care services. People with low income are sicker more often and die prematurely.[9] Income inequality refers to the unequal distribution of income in a population, and it is seen among individuals and groups of individuals. Because of the effect of income on health, income inequality is becoming a problem throughout the world, including in the United States.[10] It is known that a person's health is often poorer in a population with a low average income regardless of the person's own income. The growing inequality in income has been accompanied by inequality in wealth.[11] It is also known that as income decreases, a person's health declines, and vice versa.[12]

Income level has a direct and long-lasting effect on health. The effect of income has been shown to have an effect on health as long as fifteen years later.[13] Income inequality influences chronic disease, which takes many years to cause

FIGURE 9.1: U.S. poverty rates, 1966 to 2005

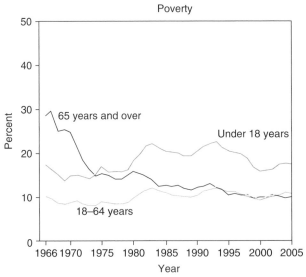

Source: CND/NCHS, *Health, United States, 2009*, Figure 4. Data from the U.S. Census Bureau.

symptoms, especially as it relates to increased mortality with heart disease. In fact, it was found that in poorer populations, the risk of death from heart disease was higher than in other populations. This was due to a higher BMI, a higher percentage of the population having hypertension, and lack of exercise.[14]

Figure 9.1 presents poverty rates in the United States from 1996 to 2005. The overall poverty rates have decreased for all Americans, with the exception of people younger than eighteen years. This group has experienced an increase in poverty since 1996, with the rate decreasing slightly the past few years. The group of people who need the most health care services, those older than sixty-five years, have a lower poverty rate today than in 1966. With Medicare paying for the health care of people older than sixty-five, they have more money for other life needs.

The relationship between income and health is dependent on income inequality. In developing countries, there are few wealthy people, the rest are poor, and the effect of income on health is pronounced. In the United States, most of the income and money belong to a small percentage of the people. However, there is a large middle class in this country, so the income is better distributed than in developing countries. The federally supported Medicare and Medicaid programs have helped to reduce the effect of income equality on health.

When the effect of income inequality was studied among African Americans in the United States, it was found to be related to higher mortality rates from coronary heart disease, malignant neoplasms, homicide, and infant mortality.[15] Income inequality has also been shown to be a risk factor for coronary heart disease. This effect is related in part to psychological conditions that may be caused by income equality. Depression is known to increase the risk of coronary heart disease, and it has been linked in some cases to income inequality.[16]

Income inequality has been shown to be related to low birth weight in infants. There is a greater chance of low-birth-weight and preterm births among people who live in poverty. The race of the mother is an important risk factor, with higher risk in minority women.[17]

Children who live in urban areas are affected by income inequality. Less than 50 percent of children with asthma who live in urban areas are treated by a physician, with Mexican Americans at the lowest percentage. Slightly more than 50 percent of the children who are treated by physicians receive the needed testing and treatment. This shows that income inequality has a negative effect on children with asthma: these children do not receive the needed care to manage their disease.[18]

Further studies have indicated that income inequality affects screening and testing for chronic diseases in adults. For example, people in lower socioeconomic groups are less likely to be screened for colon cancer. In fact, only one half of adults receive screening as described by national guidelines. The same is true for breast cancer screening in low-income Mexican American women. Those women who did not have repeated mammograms were unaware of the fatal effects of breast cancer and the importance of screening.[19]

Socioeconomic Factors and Health

It is becoming more obvious that the socioeconomic factors in childhood have a lifelong effect on the health of adults. This is the situation with infection with hepatitis B, the risk of liver cancer, and environmental lead exposure. In addition to what happens in childhood, socioeconomic factors have a cumulative effect on health throughout life.[20] This cumulative effect increases the risk of specific diseases developing.[21] People who have low educational attainment (for example, did not graduate from high school) have a greater chance of having a low-income job and working in an occupation with a high risk of toxic exposures.[22]

Coronary artery disease is an illness that develops throughout a person's life. Lifestyle behaviors throughout life have a direct influence on the development of coronary heart disease. The symptoms of coronary heart disease are seen in adults, but one of its major causes, atherosclerosis, begins much earlier in life. Fatty deposits are found in arterial linings of children.[23] During autopsies of young men who die from homicides, lesions of the coronary artery are frequent findings.[24]

Diabetes mellitus is another disease that is affected by socioeconomic position. Diabetes is common in most industrialized countries, but it is unevenly distributed in the population. The majority of people who have diabetes are in lower socioeconomic groups.[25] The effect of socioeconomic position is that prevention and treatment services are either not used or not available to most people with diabetes. In addition, people with lower levels of education often lack the understanding of the symptoms and management of diabetes.[26] Access to quality of care is adversely affected by socioeconomic status, which leads to higher rates of sickness and death in diabetic persons of low socioeconomic status.[27]

How and why does low socioeconomic position have such a negative effect on the health of people with diabetes? One reason is that people in low socioeconomic groups usually have poorer physical and mental health. In low socioeconomic groups, higher rates of smoking, lower rates of physical activity, and lower rates of self-monitoring of blood glucose levels are seen.[28]

People in higher socioeconomic groups have better health outcomes from treatment of all diseases due to several factors. First, these people have greater access to more health care providers. They also have greater access to a higher quality of care due either to health insurance or their personal ability to pay.[29] Insured people with diabetes have a three times greater chance of receiving high-quality care than those without health insurance.[30] People with health insurance receive more annual foot and eye examinations and have a lower incidence of circulation problems in their extremities and diabetic eye diseases.[31]

In addition to influencing chronic diseases, society has an effect on infectious diseases. The relationship between social determinants and HIV/AIDS is complex. HIV/AIDS can be considered a social disease because whether a person develops the disease and spreads it in a population depends on the behavior and exposure of others.[32] Social networks are important in the treatment and management of HIV/AIDS; they can influence health outcomes both directly and indirectly.[33] At the same time, social networks have also been linked to the pattern of HIV infection.[34] With HIV/AIDS, people in social networks are at risk or are HIV infected. This is a case where social networks can be both beneficial and detrimental to health outcomes.[35]

Low socioeconomic status has an effect on HIV/AIDS transmission because of varying rates of illicit drug use and condom usage. People in lower socioeconomic groups are more likely to use illicit drugs and share needles. This group of the population is also less likely to use condoms to prevent disease spread.[36]

Major mental disorders are affected by socioeconomic position. The incidence and prevalence rates of depression are higher in lower socioeconomic groups.[37] The prevalence rate of panic, phobias, and anxiety disorder is higher in people from lower social classes.[38] Low educational level is a risk factor for social phobia and obsessive-compulsive disorder.[39]

As discussed earlier in this chapter, substance abuse is affected by social determinants. Tobacco, alcohol, and illicit drug use has been shown to have a negative effect on the quality and quantity of life and on societal costs.[40] Poor grades in school, low household income, low levels of maternal education, parental smoking, and living in inner-city areas are associated with teenaged cigarette smoking.[41] Alcohol use in teenagers is associated with parental alcohol and substance abuse.[42] Social networks have an influence on whether people begin to smoke. Social networks in which there are poor relationships between parents and children, low parental educational attainment, and parental substance use are major risk factors for smoking and alcohol use in teenagers.[43]

Illicit drug usage has been studied to determine the effect of social determinants. Marijuana use has been shown to be related to drug use in social networks.[44] Peer drug use is also a risk factor for marijuana use in teenagers.[45] In addition, living in urban and inner-city areas has been shown to be associated with marijuana use.[46]

The Built Environment

The *built environment*—the manufactured physical structures and infrastructure of communities—has been linked to health and disease, both physical and mental. Today it is understood that the way the built environment has been designed is related to many public health concerns, including obesity, cardiovascular disease, diabetes, asthma, injury, depression, violence, and social inequities.

Research has shown that physical and mental health problems are related to the built environment and that there are health benefits from sustainable communities. People who come into contact with the natural environment have been shown to experience health benefits. Lower socioeconomic status communities usually have limited access to quality housing, outdoor facilities, and healthy food sources; inequities in low-income housing; high population densities; and higher rates of respiratory tract disease, developmental disorders, chronic illness, and mental illness.[47]

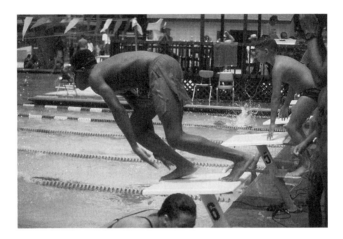

Place has health impacts that include physical, psychological, social, spiritual, and esthetic outcomes. Opportunities exist for targeting public health problems as they relate to aspects of the built environment (nature contact, buildings, public spaces, and urban form). Research in this area is expected to lead to new opportunities in understanding how the built environment can be designed to improve health.[48]

It has been common to house poor people in dense, large urban developments, typically public housing; however, this arrangement causes several health problems, including stress. People living in low-income neighborhoods are affected both physically and mentally. In fact, one research study learned that parents who were moved from low-income neighborhoods realized significant reductions in stress. In addition, boys who moved to less poor neighborhoods reported less depressive and dependency problems.[49]

The built environment is thought to be one of the many causes of overweight and obesity in children and adolescents. Children and adults who live in neighborhoods that have easy access to convenience stores have the greatest chance of becoming overweight or obese. It was found that if men and women older than fifty-five years live in an affluent neighborhood, they are less likely to be obese.[50]

The built environment affects physical activity. The level of greenness (parks and open green spaces) has been found to have a positive effect on health.

Children living in areas with higher levels of greenness have lower BMI scores and are healthier. This is due to the chance of more physical activity and time spent outdoors.[51]

The health benefits of walking have been known for many years, and this was highlighted in the U.S. Surgeon General's report on physical activity.[52] The report stated that lack of physical activity was an important disease risk factor. The built environment has a direct influence on whether people participate in physical activity, including walking. Local walking patterns are influenced by neighborhood design.[53] Interestingly, people who live in urban and inner-city areas are more likely to walk because of the heavy traffic flow, the lack of trees, and the availability of sidewalks.[54]

How does transportation within the built environment affect social determinants and health? The World Health Organization has stated that transportation is an important factor for health.[55] It is beginning to be understood that automobile use has a negative influence on social capital and health.[56] So a side effect of the industrialization and development of the United States is an adverse effect on health.[57] Automobile usage can be associated with increased levels of air pollution, urban sprawl, and the increase in the prevalence of obesity.[58]

SOCIAL CAPITAL

Social capital refers to community improvement, social networking, civic engagement, personal recreation, and other activities that establish social connections between people and groups.

The built environment can directly affect the amount of time for family gatherings, recreation, and community involvement. The effect of the built environment on social capital can be either positive or negative.

Source: Centers for Disease Control and Prevention. Healthy Places: http://www.cdc.gov/HEALTHYPLACES/healthtopics/social.htm.

Figure 9.2 shows overweight and obesity rates in the United States from 1960 to 2004. During this twenty-five-year period, the prevalence rate of overweight and obesity has significantly increased in all age groups. The rate of overweight alone in the twenty- to seventy-four-years age group has remained

FIGURE 9.2: Prevalence rate of overweight and obesity, United States, 1960 to 2004

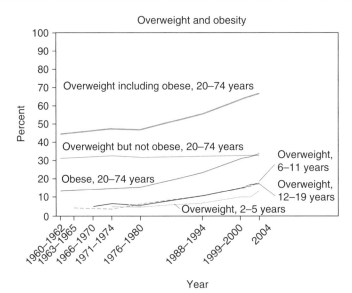

Source: CND/NCHS, *Health, United States, 2009*, Figure 7. Data from the National Health Examination Survey and the National Health and Nutrition Examination Survey.

the same. The troubling finding is the increase in overweight in the younger age groups. As was mentioned earlier in this chapter, socioeconomic factors in childhood have a lasting, lifelong effect. This is a bad omen for future obesity prevalence in adults.

Summary

Society and social conditions have been linked to health and disease. Where and how (individual lifestyles) people live are directly related to disease. Many chronic diseases (for example, heart disease) are linked to lifestyles. The branch of epidemiology called social epidemiology studies the influence of society on health and disease. This study is done by evaluating social determinants, which include socioeconomic status and income. Income inequality has been shown to be one of the explanations for disease and health disparities in the United States.

Where people live has been studied for some time to evaluate its effect on health. The study of the built environment has resulted in many interesting findings. The built environment affects physical activity. If where people live is characterized by parks and sidewalks, then physical activity is high. For people who live in suburban areas without sidewalks and where there is an increased dependency on automobiles, physical activity is low. Many chronic diseases and conditions, including obesity, are directly affected by lack of physical activity.

Key Terms

Built environment, 185　　　　　Social epidemiology, 180

Income inequality, 181

Chapter Exercises

This chapter has presented the effect of social determinants and the built environment on health, both physical and mental. The chapter exercises will focus on how social determinants and the built environment can affect your daily life.

1. Create a log of the amount of miles and time you spend using a motorized vehicle (automobile, truck, van, sports-utility vehicle, or motorcycle) for the next two weeks.
2. Create a walking log of your daily activities for the next two weeks. In this log, record your walking starting points and destinations, the approximate distance, and the time spent walking. Include recreational walking.
3. Using the information in the two newly created logs, analyze the information to determine
   a. average amount of time you spend in a motorized vehicle each day,
   b. average distance (in miles) you travel in a motorized vehicle each day,
   c. average amount of time you spend walking each day, and
   d. average distance you walk each day.

4. Write a report discussing your logs (include the logs as appendices) and discuss whether or not you feel that your physical activity can be improved to positively influence your health.

Chapter Review

1. A person's risk is not related to the place where they live. True or False?
2. Social epidemiology
   a. developed as a science in the eighteenth century.
   b. studies the effect of social determinants on health and disease.
   c. does not use traditional epidemiological information.
   d. none of the above.
3. Socioeconomic position
   a. is an indicator of the social effects on health.
   b. combines many characteristics, including income and educational level.
   c. has been suggested as a cause of increased risk for coronary disease.
   d. is the same as social class.
   e. all of the above.
4. Income inequality has been shown to affect health and disease. True or False?
5. Poverty rates in the United States for people aged sixty-five years and older
   a. have remained unchanged since the 1960s.
   b. have increased since the 1960s.
   c. have decreased since the 1960s.
   d. none of the above.
6. People in higher socioeconomic groups have better health. True or False?
7. The following diseases are affected by socioeconomic position:
   a. diabetes
   b. coronary artery disease
   c. mental disorders
   d. all of the above.
   e. none of the above.
8. People who live in lower socioeconomic neighborhoods have poorer health outcomes. True or False?
9. Where people live can affect
   a. physical health.
   b. psychological health.
   c. spiritual health.
   d. social outcomes.

 e. all of the above.

 f. none of the above.

10. The percentage of the people in the United States who are overweight or obese has

 a. remained unchanged since the 1960s.

 b. increased since the 1960s.

 c. decreased since the 1960s.

 d. none of the above.

SCREENING FOR DISEASE

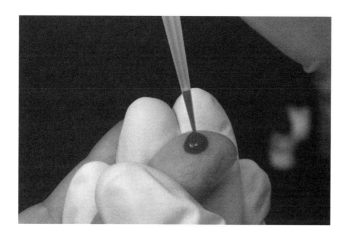

LEARNING OBJECTIVES

On completing this chapter, you will be able to

Discuss prevention of disease
Define validity and reliability
Define sensitivity and specificity
Define predictive values of a positive and negative screening test result

Prevention and Epidemiology

Preventing disease is more important than treating disease. In fact, it has been estimated that half of all deaths each year are preventable.[1] Prevention of disease is a part of epidemiology because preventive methods are guided by epidemiological principles. Prevention activities can be categorized as being either *primary*, *secondary*, or *tertiary*, based on the progression of a disease process from being free of disease all the way to showing the effects of clinical disease, with its associated disability and possibility of death.[2,3]

Primary prevention is concerned with eliminating the risk factors for a disease. Primary prevention intends to avert the development of disease before it occurs by preventing the development of new cases of a disease. So primary prevention decreases the incidence rate of a disease. Health promotion is an example of primary prevention. Hospitals often sponsor health fairs and go to area schools to discuss health and disease factors. These hospital-sponsored wellness fairs are done to educate communities about potential risk factors and to increase community awareness of available hospital services. Another example of primary prevention is nutrition counseling for children. Because the early onset of coronary artery disease has been related to elevated cholesterol levels in children, designing and implementing lower-fat pediatric diets should result in the elimination of a major risk factor for coronary artery disease. Other examples of primary prevention include the use of automobile seat belts, condom use, skin protection from the harmful effects of sunlight, and tobacco-use cessation programs.

Secondary prevention focuses on early detection and treatment of a disease, especially when symptoms of a disease are not noticeable (this is known as *subclinical disease*). Secondary prevention tries to reduce the burden of existing disease after it has developed, with emphasis on preventing disease complications. Secondary prevention activities are aimed at slowing the progression of disease, eliminating disease, and limiting adverse effects of disease, such as disability. If secondary prevention is successful in eliminating disease, then the prevalence rate will decrease. An example of secondary prevention is periodic cholesterol testing in children with a family history of coronary heart disease. Family history is a risk factor that cannot be changed, so early detection can be accomplished through periodic testing. Other examples of secondary prevention include periodic testing of cholesterol levels in adults, periodic breast and prostate examinations, and Pap smears, because these tests focus on the early detection of disease.

Tertiary prevention attempts to eliminate or reduce the disability that is associated with advanced disease. Tertiary prevention tries to help people who have suffered irreversible effects of a disease to reach optimal health status. Tertiary prevention involves rehabilitation and limitation of disability. Physical activity for heart attack patients is an example of tertiary prevention. Physical therapy programs for stroke patients and individuals who have experienced traumatic injuries are another example, as is inpatient respiratory therapy.

Screening

The purpose of screening is to identify disease early in its development so it can be stopped or altered and have less effect on people. Screening is done when a disease causes a high rate of death or illness, a test (or tests) are at hand that can detect a disease in its early development, and an effective treatment (or treatments) is easily available.[4] A screening test should have the following characteristics:

- It is simple and easy to do.

- It is quick to do.

- It is inexpensive, especially when screening a large number of people.

- It is safe, and people are not harmed by the screening test.

- It is acceptable to the people in the population.[5]

In real-life situations, diseases are chosen to be screened if there is a long time between a disease developing and symptoms showing (called the presymptomatic phase). These diseases can be detected early, and treatment can be begun with a good chance of stopping the harmful effects. Without screening, when these diseases are discovered (because symptoms are not apparent), it may be too late to provide helpful treatment.

The *yield of a screening test* is defined as the number of people who are identified who may otherwise not be detected. The yield of a screening test is important because it quantifies the number of people who will have a better outcome from treatment of a disease because of early detection. The yield is one way to evaluate the effectiveness of a screening test, but the total number of screening tests must be included in the evaluation. For example, for every new case of breast cancer that is detected by screening, 170 women must be screened.

An example of the yield of a screening test is the Prostate, Lung, Colorectal, Ovarian Cancer (PLCO) trial that was begun in 1993. A total of 38,350 men were screened for prostate cancer by an annual PSA blood test and digital rectal exams. During the screening, 14 percent of the men had abnormal results from one or both of the screening tests. Of these men, 31 percent had a prostate biopsy. Almost 2 percent of the men in the study were diagnosed as having cancer by a prostate biopsy, which is the yield of the prostate screening tests.[6]

The yield of a screening test depends on its *sensitivity* and *specificity*. A good screening test will have high sensitivity and high specificity. High sensitivity indicates that the screening test correctly identifies the small proportion of screened people who actually have the disease. High specificity indicates there are few false-positive results, thereby eliminating the need for additional treatment and testing.

Accuracy of Screening Tests

Accuracy is an indicator of a screening test's performance. Accuracy is defined as "the condition of being true, correct, or exact." Accuracy can be thought of as how often a test correctly identifies people who have a disease and others who do not have a disease. The measurement for accuracy is called *validity*. In addition to accuracy, it is important to measure the precision of a screening test. This is done by a measurement called *reliability*.[7] These measurements will be discussed later after the opposite—error—is presented.

Error is an important concern and major worry of screening tests. *Error* can be defined as any difference between an observed screening test result and the actual (or true) result. If a screening test identifies someone as having a disease when they don't, this is error. If a screening test measures high blood pressure when the person has normal blood pressure, this is error.

Error is classified in two ways: random and systematic. *Random error,* also called *chance error* or *sampling error,* is termed random because the errors are unpredictable and can happen whenever measurements are taken. They can be caused by biological differences in the people screened and unpredictable fluctuations in the readings of a measurement apparatus. *Systematic error,* also known as *bias,* is the error that is not random. Systematic error happens when there are problems with measuring instruments or the environment that can affect the measurements. Systematic error can be caused by selection bias, which is when people choose or are convinced to undergo a screening test or by the tester or the test makeup. For example, when test tubes are incorrectly labeled, systematic error results.

Validity

Validity is the ability of a test to produce a true measure. The truth is what validity measures. Validity is quantified by the four parameters: sensitivity, specificity, and predictive values (of positive and negative test results). Of course, a well-accepted confirmatory test that identifies the true measure is needed to verify and quantify validity. These confirmatory tests include blood tests and biopsies.

To understand the parameters of validity, reviewing a 2×2 contingency table is helpful (Table 10.1). The table consists of two columns that represent the true disease status (the person has disease or not) and two rows that represent the test results (the person tests positive or negative for the disease). The top left cell, labeled a, shows the number of people with the disease who are correctly identified by the screening test result. Because the people in cell a truly have the disease and the screening test result is positive for the disease, they are called *true positives* (TP). The top right cell, labeled b, shows the number of people who do not have the disease but are incorrectly identified by the screening test results as having the disease; they are called *false positives* (FP). The bottom left cell, labeled c, shows the number of people who have the disease but the screening test does not identify the disease. Because these people in cell c have the disease but the screening test falsely identifies them as being negative for the disease, they are called *false negatives* (FN). The bottom right cell, labeled d, shows the number of people who do not have the disease and the screening test correctly identifies them as not having the disease; the screening test result is called *true negative* (TN).

TABLE 10.1: 2×2 Contingency Table

	Disease	No Disease	Total
Test result is positive for the disease	a TP	b FP	$a + b$
Test result is negative for the disease	c FN	d TN	$c + d$
Total	$a + c$	$b + d$	$a + b + c + d$

True positives (TP) = people who have the disease, and the screening test result is positive for the disease; false positives (FP) = people who do not have the disease, but they have been falsely identified as having the disease by a positive test result; false negatives (FN) = people who have the disease, but the screening test has falsely identified them as not having the disease by the negative test result; and true negatives (TN) = people who do not have the disease, and the screening test has a negative test result.

The goal when performing a screening test (and any other test) is to have as many true test results as possible, which are seen in the number of true positives and true negatives. This is done by limiting (and hopefully eliminating) the number of incorrect test results, which are seen in the number of false positives and false negatives. Sensitivity, specificity, and the predictive values of positive and negative test results (called predictive values) are used to measure achievement of this goal. Sensitivity, which measures the number of people with the disease that the test correctly identifies as having the disease, is defined as the ability of a test to correctly identify those people who have a disease. Sensitivity is also known as the true-positive ratio (TP ratio) because it is equal to the ratio of the true positive results in those people in cell a to the number of people with the disease (total number of people in the left column, or the disease column). The total number of people in the disease column is calculated by $a + c$. The TP ratio is calculated by dividing the number of people in cell a by the total number of people in the left (disease) column, or $a/(a + c)$. Table 10.2 shows the calculation for the sensitivity.

Specificity, which measures the number of people without disease that the screening test correctly identifies as having negative results for the disease, can be defined as the ability of a test to correctly identify those individuals who do not have a disease. Specificity is also known as the true-negative (TN) ratio because it is equal to the ratio of the TNs, cell d (Table 10.3), to the number of people without the disease (total number of people in the right column, or no-disease column). The total number of people in the no-disease column is calculated by $b + d$. The TN ratio is calculated by dividing the number of people in cell d by the total number of people in the right (no-disease) column, or $(d/(b + d)$.

Sensitivity and specificity can be expressed as either a percentage or as a probability. Probabilities are positive numbers that are between 0 and 1. So sensitivity can be written as 96 percent or 0.96. A perfect test will have a sensitiv-

TABLE 10.2: Sensitivity: True-Positive Ratio

	Disease	No-Disease	Total
Test result is positive for the disease	a TP		
Test result is negative for the disease	c FN		
Total	$a + c$		

Sensitivity = TP/Disease Column Total = $a/(a + c)$.

TABLE 10.3: Specificity: True-Negative Ratio

	Disease	No Disease	Total
Test result is positive for the disease		b	
		FP	
Test result is negative for the disease		d	
		TN	
Total		b + d	

Specificity = TN/No Disease Column Total = $d/(b + d)$.

TABLE 10.4: False-Positive (FP) Ratio

	Disease	No Disease	Total
Test result is positive for the disease		b	
		FP	
Test result is negative for the disease		d	
		TN	
Total		b + d	

FP Ratio = FP/No Disease Column Total = $b/(b + d)$ = 1–specificity.

ity of 1 (100 percent of the time, the test will correctly identify people who have the disease) and a specificity of 1 (100 percent of the time, the test will correctly identify people who do not have the disease). This means that the test would identify those people with and without the disease correctly every time the test was performed. The closer the sensitivity is to 1, the more accurate the test is in identifying people with a disease, and the closer the specificity is to 1, the more accurate the test is in identifying people without a disease.

In addition to sensitivity and specificity, the 2×2 contingency tables can be used to gather more information about the screening tests. The 2×2 table can be used to calculate the complements of sensitivity and specificity, which are the *false-negative ratio* (FN ratio) and the *false-positive ratio* (FP ratio). *Complements* are two numbers that added up to one. The columns of the 2×2 table are used to calculate the complements. The FN ratio and the TP ratio (sensitivity) add up to one and are complements. The FP ratio and the TN ratio (specificity) add up to one and are complements. In other words, the FN ratio is equal to 1-sensitivity, and the FP ratio is equal to 1-specificity.

The calculation of the FP ratio is shown in Table 10.4. The FP ratio is equal to the ratio of FPs, cell *b*, to the number of people without the disease (total number of people in the right column, or no disease column). The total number

TABLE 10.5: False–Negative (FN) Ratio

	Disease	No Disease	Total
Test result is positive for the disease	a TP		
Test result is negative for the disease	c FN		
Total	a + c		

FN Ratio = FN/Disease Column Total = $c/(a + c)$ = 1–sensitivity.

TABLE 10.6: Validity Calculation Example

Physical Exam Result	Breast Cancer	No Breast Cancer	Totals
Positive for breast cancer	a 1,800	b 800	a + b 2,600
Negative for breast cancer	c 700	d 4,200	c + d 4,900
Totals	a + c 2,500	b + d 5,000	a + b + c + d 7,500

of people in the no-disease column is calculated by $b + d$. The FP ratio is calculated by dividing the number of people in cell b by the total number of people in the right (no-disease column, or $b/(b + d)$. As mentioned above, you can calculate the specificity and then determine the FP ratio by using 1-specificity.

The calculation of the FN ratio is shown in Table 10.5. The FN ratio is equal to the ratio of FNs, cell c, to the number of people with the disease (total number of people in the left column, or disease column). The total number of people in the disease column is calculated by $a + c$. The FN ratio is calculated by dividing the number of people in cell c by the total number of people in the left (disease) column, or $c/(a + c)$. Another way is to calculate the sensitivity, then determine the FN ratio using 1-sensitivity.

Table 10.6 shows the result of a physical examination that was used as a screening test of women for breast cancer in a public health clinic in a large metropolitan area. During a twelve-month period, 7,500 women were screened for breast cancer. Of these women, 2,600 had a biopsy confirmation of breast cancer. The remaining 4,900 women of the same age category and race did not have cancer. When the screening physical examination was done, a positive test result for cancer (a mass found by the physical examination) resulted in 1,800 women who had biopsy-confirmed breast cancer and 800 women who did not have cancer. A 2×2 contingency table can be used to understand the parameters of validity. The 1,800 women with the positive screening test result who have cancer had true–positive results and are in the cell labeled a. The 800 women who do not have cancer but had a positive screening test result, called false-positive, are in the cell labeled b. The total number of women with breast cancer, 2,500, is the left column total. The total number of women who do not have breast cancer is the right column total.

Following the notion of complements, the number of FNs, which are placed in the cell labeled c, is equal to the total number of women with biopsy-confirmed breast cancer, 2,500, minus the number of TPs. The number of FNs is 2,500 minus 1,800, or 700. Again following the notion of complements, the number of TNs, which is placed in the cell labeled d, is equal to the total number of women who do not have cancer (5,000) minus the number of FPs. The number of TNs is 5,000 minus 800, or 4,200.

The sensitivity and specificity can be calculated using the columns of the 2×2 table (see Tables 10.7 and 10.8). The sensitivity is the ratio of TPs to the total number of women who have cancer. The sensitivity is calculated as

TABLE 10.7: Validity Calculation Example: Sensitivity

Physical Exam Result	Breast Cancer	No Breast Cancer	Totals
Positive for breast cancer	a 1,800		
Negative for breast cancer	c 700		
Totals	$a + c$ 2,500		

Sensitivity = TP/Disease Column Total = $a/(a + c)$ = 1,800/2,500 = 0.72.

TABLE 10.8: Validity Calculation Example: Specificity

Physical Exam Result	Breast Cancer	No Breast Cancer	Totals
Positive for breast cancer		b 800	
Negative for breast cancer		d 4,200	
Totals		$b + d$ 5,000	

Specificity = TN/No Disease Column Total = $d/(b + d)$ = 4,200/5,000 = 0.84.

TABLE 10.9: Validity Calculation Example: FN Ratio

Physical Exam Result	Breast Cancer	No Breast Cancer	Totals
Positive for breast cancer	a 1,800		
Negative for breast cancer	c 700		
Totals	a + c 2,500		

FN Ratio = FN/Disease Column Total = $c/(a + c)$ = 700/2,500 = 0.28.

TABLE 10.10: Validity Calculation Example: FP Ratio

Physical Exam Result	Breast Cancer	No Breast Cancer	Totals
Positive for breast cancer		b 800	
Negative for breast cancer		d 4,200	
Totals		b + d 5,000	

FP Ratio = FP/No Disease Column Total = $b/(b + d)$ = 800/5,000 = 0.16.

$a/(a+c)$. The sensitivity of the screening physical examination is 1,800 divided by 2,500, or 0.72. The specificity is the ratio of TNs to the total number of women who do not have cancer. The specificity is calculated as $d/c + d$. The specificity of the screening physical examination is 4,200 divided by 5,000, or 0.84.

Tables 10.9 and 10.10 present the calculation of the FN and FP ratios using the above example. The FN ratio is equal to the ratio of FNs to the total number of women who have cancer. The FN ratio is calculated as $c/(a+c)$. The FN ratio of the screening physical examination is 700 divided by 2,500, or 0.28. The FP ratio is equal to the ratio of FPs to the total number of women who do not have cancer. The FP ratio is calculated as $b/(b + d)$. The FP ratio of the screening physical examination is 800 divided by 5,000, or 0.16.

Believe it or not, the 2×2 contingency table contains even more information about the accuracy of a screening test. In addition to the information that we can get from the columns of the 2×2 table, the rows are helpful in understanding the validity of a screening test. The top row contains the number of people who have a positive screening test result. These people are identified by the screening test as having the disease. The bottom row contains the number of

TABLE 10.11: Predictive Value of a Positive Test Result (PV+)

	Disease	No Disease	Total
Test result positive for the disease	a TP	b FP	a + b
Test result negative for the disease Total			

PV+ = TP/Positive Test Result for the Disease Row Total = $a/(a + b)$.

TABLE 10.12: Predictive Value of a Negative Test Result (PV–)

	Disease	No Disease	Total
Test result positive for the disease			
Test result negative for the disease	c FN	d TN	c + d
Total			

PV– = TN/Negative Test Result for the Disease Row Total = $d/(c + d)$.

people who have a negative screening test result and are those people who the screening test identifies as not having the disease.

The rows are used to calculate the predictive values of a positive and negative test result (Table 10.11). The top row information is used to calculate the predictive value of a positive test result (PV+), and the bottom row is used to calculate the predictive value of a negative test result (PV–). The PV+ is equal to the ratio of the number of TPs, cell *a*, to the number of people who have a positive test result (total number in the top row, or positive test result row). The total number in the row is *a* + *b*. The PV+ is calculated by dividing the number in cell *a* by the total number in the top (positive test result) row, or $a/(a + b)$.

The PV– is calculated using the bottom row, or the negative test result row (Table 10.12). The PV– is equal to the ratio of TNs, cell *d*, to the number in the bottom row, or negative test result row. The total number in the bottom row is calculated by *c* + *d*. The PV– is calculated by dividing the number of TNs in cell *d* by the total number of people in the bottom (negative test result) row, or $d/(c + d)$.

An example of calculating the predictive values of a positive and negative test result is the above-mentioned physical screening examination. The predictive values of the physical screening examination can be calculated by using the rows of the 2×2 tables (see Tables 10.13 and 10.14). The total number of women in the top row equals the number of TPs plus the number of FPs, 1,800 plus

TABLE 10.13: Validity Calculation Example: PV+

Physical Exam Result	Breast Cancer	No Breast Cancer	Totals
Positive for breast cancer	a 1,800	b 800	a + b 2,600
Negative for breast cancer			
Totals			

PV+ = TP/Positive Test Result for Breast Cancer Disease Row Total = $a/(a + b)$ = 1,800/2,600 = 0.69.

TABLE 10.14: Validity Calculation Example: PV−

Physical Exam Result	Breast Cancer	No Breast Cancer	Totals
Positive for breast cancer			
Negative for breast cancer	c 700	d 4,200	c + d 4,900
Totals			

PV+ = TN/Negative Test Result for Breast Cancer = $d/(c + d)$ = 4,200/4,900 = 0.86.

800, or 2,600. The total number of women in the bottom row equals the number of FNs plus the number of TNs, 700 plus 4,200, or 4,900. The PV+ is the ratio of the TPs to the total number of positive test results. The PV+ is calculated as $a/(a + b)$. The PV+ for the physical screening examination is 1,800 divided by 2,600, or 0.69. The PV− is the ratio of TNs to the total number of negative test results. The PV− is calculated as $d/(c + d)$. The PV− for the physical screening examination is 4,200 divided by 4,900, or 0.86.

Prevalence and Validity

The *prevalence rate* is the number of current cases of disease in the population at a given time. The prevalence rate has an influence on some of the validity parameters. Thus is due to the impact of the number of people in the population on the ability of the screening test to correctly identify people who have and those who do not have the disease.

The ability of a test to correctly identify whether people have a disease (sensitivity) and whether they do not have a disease (specificity) is not influenced by the prevalence rate. But the predictive values of a positive and negative test are directly affected. What happens is if the prevalence rate of a disease increases in a population, the PV+ increases. When the prevalence rate of a disease decreases, the PV+ decreases. So the prevalence rate and the PV+ change in the same direction, or they are directly and positively correlated.

If the prevalence rate of a disease increases, the PV− decreases. When the prevalence rate of a disease decreases, the PV− increases. What is happening is that the prevalence rate of a disease and the PV− change in the opposite direction, or they are directly and negatively correlated.

One explanation for this relationship is that if many people in a population have a disease, then the chance that the screening test will correctly identify them is high. If few people in a population have the disease, then the chance that the screening test will identify them is low. Additionally, if there are many people in the population with a disease then the chance that the screening test result will be positive for the disease is high. Conversely, if only a few people in a population have a disease, then the chance that the screening test result will be negative for the disease is high.

Reliability

After it is known that a screening test is valid, next it is important to know if the test is reliable. Reliability is concerned with whether the screening test can repeat the outcomes. Reliability is defined as the degree to which repeated testing results in the same results, on the same person, under the same conditions. Reliability is often referred to as "precision," "reproducibility," and "repeatability." Reliability is concerned with whether a blood pressure cuff, which is used to measure a person's blood pressure, will give the same results when the reading is repeated over a short period.

Differences in measurements are a common concern, and they can be caused by many factors. First, differences may be caused by biological differences among persons. Second, they may be caused by physical or mental changes in people as a result of therapeutic interventions (medications and the like). Third, the differences may be caused by physical changes in people over the course of time (for example, blood pressure measurements are different in the same individual in the morning and at night).

Differences in measurements may also be caused by factors that do not involve the people undergoing the screening but involve the equipment and tester. Laboratory equipment and testing machinery may be correctly calibrated and the testing method may be properly performed, but the interpretation of the results may cause variation. When screening tests involve someone observing

TABLE 10.15: Reliability Index

		Observer 1		
		Test Result Positive for Disease (T+)	Test Result Negative for Disease (T−)	Total
Observer 2	T+	a	b	$a + b$
	T−	c	d	$c + d$
	Total	$a + c$	$b + d$	$a + b + c + d$

Reliability Index = Total Cells in Agreement/Total Number of observations = $(a + d)/(a + b + c + d)$.

a test result (for example, someone reading chest x-rays), variation may be caused by differences in the people making the observations (this is called "observer-based variation"). In fact, physicians often interpret physical and laboratory test results differently, with disagreement as to which test results are negative or positive for a disease. *Interobserver variation* happens when measurement results differ between two different observers. *Intraobserver variation* happens when the same observer comes up with different measurement results at different times.

There is a way to understand and measure both interobserver and intraobserver variations: a *reliability index* can be used. Because different people often disagree, this index (which is known as the overall proportion of agreement) is used to identify levels of acceptable variation. The index measures the degree to which two observers' measurements agree with each other or one observer's measurements agree at different times.

A 2×2 contingency table demonstrates the calculation of the reliability index (see Table 10.15). The columns and rows contain information on the interpretation of the test results by two observers (or one observer at two different times). The left column shows when observer 1 identifies a test result as positive (T+). The right column shows when observer 1 identifies a test result as negative (T−). The top row shows when observer 2 identifies a test result as positive (T+). The bottom row shows when observer 2 identifies a test result as negative (T−).

The top left cell, labeled *a*, shows the number of times observers 1 and 2 agree that there is a T+. The top right cell, labeled *b*, shows the number of times the two observers disagree, with observer 1 identifying a T− and observer 2 identifying a T+. The bottom left cell, labeled *c*, shows the number of times the two observers disagree, with observer 1 identifying a T+ and observer 2 identifying a T−. The bottom right cell, labeled *d*, shows the number of times the two observers agree that there is a T−. The reliability index is the ratio of the total

TABLE 10.16: Reliability Index Example

		T+	T–	Total
Observer 2	T+	a	b	a + b
		25	18	43
	T–	c	d	c + d
		20	137	157
	Total	a + c	b + d	a + b + c + d
		45	155	200

Reliability index = $(a + d)/(a + b + c + d) = (25 + 137)/200 = 162/200 = 0.81$.

number of times that both observers agree $(a + d)$ to the total number of observations $(a + b + c + d)$. The reliability index is calculated by dividing the times that both observers agree $(a + d)$ by the total number of observations $(a + b + c + d)$, or $(a + d)/(a + b + c + d)$.

Reliability Index Example

An example of the calculation of the reliability index is presented in Table 10.16. The example shows the situation when two radiologists review 200 chest x-rays for abnormal lung tissue. Both radiologists review the same 200 x-rays collected from 200 different people. Of the 200 x-rays reviewed, both radiologists agreed that there was abnormal lung tissue on 25 x-rays (cell a), and they agreed that 137 x-rays did not show abnormal lung tissue (cell d). So out of 200 x-rays, the radiologists agreed on their review of 162 x-rays. The reliability index equals the ratio of the times the radiologists agreed ($a + d$, or 162) to the total number of x-rays reviewed ($a + b + c + d$, or 200), or 162 divided by 200, for an index of 0.81. This means that the two radiologists agree 81 percent of the time.

Summary

Screening for disease is an important aspect of public health. Screening is done in an effort to identify early stages of disease so it can be stopped or treated successfully. Screening tests are evaluated by their yield, which is the identification of people who have undetected disease and usually no symptoms of disease.

An important concern is the accuracy of screening tests. Screening tests should be correct when they either do or do not detect disease. Validity is a measurement of accuracy. Validity is determined by sensitivity, specificity, and the predictive values of positive and negative test results. A second concern is whether screening tests are reliable: do they give consistent results? The reliability index measures the test's consistency.

Key Terms

Accuracy, 196

Chance error, 196

Complements, 196

Error, 199

False negatives (FN), 197

False-negative ratio, 199

False positives (FP), 197

False-positive ratio, 199

Interobserver variation, 206

Intraobserver variation, 206

Predictive value, 193

Prevalence rate, 204

Primary prevention, 194

Random error, 196

Reliability, 196

Reliability index, 206

Sampling error, 196

Secondary prevention, 194

Sensitivity, 196

Specificity, 196

Subclinical disease, 194

Systematic error, 196

Tertiary prevention, 195

True negatives (TN), 197

True-negative ratio, 199

True positives (TP), 197

True-positive ratio, 199

Validity, 196

Yield of a screening test, 195

Chapter Exercises

In a large multihospital study, 1,500 people who have had a proven myocardial infarction (MI) were compared with 3,500 people who have not had an MI. Electrocardiography (ECG), which detects previous infarctions, was used to identify those who had an MI. An abnormal ECG result indicates a previous MI. Table 10.17 shows the results of this study.

TABLE 10.17: ECG Results

	Previous MI	No Previous MI	Totals
Abnormal ECG	1,360	525	1,885
Normal ECG	140	2,975	3,115
Totals	1,500	3,500	5,000

1. What is the number of false positives?
2. What is the sensitivity of the ECG?
3. What is the predictive value of a positive test result?
4. What is the predictive value of a negative test result?
5. Do you think that the ECG is a good screening test?

Chapter Review

1. The reliability of a screening test is
   a. the ability of the test to distinguish between people who are truly diseased and people who truly do not have a disease.
   b. the degree to which a test on the same person will give the same test result when the test is repeated.
   c. the same as validity.
   d. all of the above.
   e. none of the above.
2. The validity of a screening test is
   a. the ability of the test to distinguish between people who are truly diseased and people who truly do not have a disease.
   b. the degree to which a test on the same person will give the same test result when the test is repeated.
   c. the same as reliability.
   d. all of the above.
   e. none of the above.
3. Two radiologists independently review 100 chest x-rays. The reliability index is 0.60. This indicates that
   a. both agreed that 60 percent of the x-rays were positive for lung lesions.
   b. both agreed that 40 percent of the x-rays were positive for lung lesions.
   c. both have the same results for 60 of the 100 chest x-rays
   d. none of the above.
4. The predictive value of a positive test result is the
   a. proportion of truly diseased people who test positive for the disease.
   b. proportion of truly nondiseased people who test positive for the disease.
   c. proportion of people who are screened who are truly diseased.
   d. none of the above.
5. The sensitivity and specificity of a screening test measure
   a. reliability.
   b. validity.
   c. precision.

    d. all of the above.

    e. none of the above.

6. The sensitivity is a complement of

    a. the TN ratio.

    b. the specificity.

    c. the FP ratio.

    d. none of the above.

7. The specificity is a complement of

    a. the TN ratio.

    b. the sensitivity.

    c. the FP ratio.

    d. none of the above.

8. The yield of a screening test is

    a. the same as the reliability.

    b. the number of people who are identified who may otherwise not be detected.

    c. affected by sensitivity and specificity of the screening test.

    d. all of the above.

    e. none of the above.

9. The sensitivity of a screening test is directly affected by the prevalence rate. True or False?

10. The predictive values of a screening test are directly affected by the prevalence rate. True or False?

COMMUNITY PUBLIC HEALTH

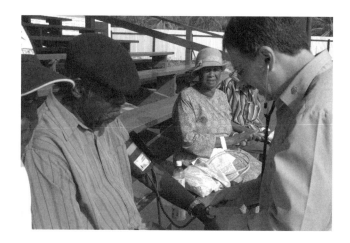

LEARNING OBJECTIVES

On completing this chapter, you will be able to

Discuss the role of community health workers
Describe the planning and evaluation process
Describe logic models and their use in evaluation
Describe examples of public health programs

Introduction

Before beginning our discussion of community public health, we must first discuss *community*. There have been many definitions of the term community, including the following by the Merriam-Webster Online dictionary: community is a unified body of people with common interests living in a particular area. Community public health has been seen as public health programs that are aimed at preventing or controlling specific diseases. Often public health policy and program development happen at a national or regional geographical level, but real public health occurs at the level of the community. In fact, the characteristics of a community have been shown to have a direct influence on public health programs.[1] Knowing this, it is important to earn the respect and collaboration of individual communities before beginning public health programs. Of course, the problem is determining who and what is the community.

In public health and epidemiology, there are common aspects of the many definitions of the term community. These aspects are location, sharing, joint action, social connections, and diversity, and a good definition of community is "a group of people with diverse characteristics who are linked by social ties, share common perspectives, and engage in joint action in geographic locations or settings."[2]

Location refers to a place that is common to all members of the community and is associated with a physical setting in which people in a community feel comfortable and safe. Sharing has a more complex and multifaceted meaning. *Sharing* refers to common interests and perceptions of the people who contribute to the feeling of community. These include values, beliefs, opinions, concerns, goals, symbols, history, comfort, familiarity, togetherness, and identity. *Joint actions* affect togetherness and identity. Examples of joint actions include working at voting polls, volunteering at public hospitals and libraries, contributing to community food banks, and neighborhood watch programs.

Social connections are the foundation of communities. *Social connections* are the interpersonal relationships of people in the community. These relationships go beyond family and friends to include neighbors and others in the community. Social connections lead to a feeling of community because people want to be associated with others whom they trust, feel comfortable with in their presence, care about, often see in the community, and grow up with and attend school together. People want to live and work with others whom they feel have common interests and challenges.

Community Health Workers

The public health system is dependent on qualified, well-educated, and dedicated workers. *Community health workers* are "community members who work almost exclusively in community settings. They serve as connectors between health care consumers and providers to promote health among groups that have traditionally lacked access to adequate health care."[3] Community health workers have been called many names, including community health advocates, lay health educators, community health representatives, community health outreach workers, and *promotoras de salud*.

What makes community health workers so successful is that they live in the communities in which they work, can easily communicate with locals, and are quickly trusted by people in the community.[4] Community health workers effectively promote health and help people in the community handle the stresses of life.[5] They establish a community-based health care system that uses social support to enhance the health care services provided by local doctors and hospitals.[6]

Seven core roles of community health workers have been identified:

1. bridging cultural mediation between communities and the health care system,

2. providing culturally appropriate and accessible health education and information,

3. assuring that people get needed services,

4. providing informal counseling and social support,

5. advocating for people and communities within the health and social service systems,

6. providing direct services (for example, basic first aid) and administering health screening tests,

7. building individual and community capacity.[7]

An example of how community health workers interact with the community is the Ohio Children's Buy-In Program.[8] This is a statewide plan that allows families living in poverty to buy public health insurance. Families enroll in this program online. Community health workers provide coaching and emotional support during the application process by staffing an online "help desk." The personal caring provided by the community health workers has helped to make this program, in its early stages, successful.

Another example involves the use of promotoras de salud in asthma treatment programs.[9] Promotoras conduct home visits and follow-up encounters with families over a three-month period in an attempt to increase asthma knowledge and quality of life by decreasing the frequency of triggering events. The promotoras evaluate changes in families' knowledge of asthma and the reduction of triggering events. The promotoras have been successful in linking families with health care providers and the school system.

Promotoras have also been used to develop healthy neighborhoods in areas of dense Latino populations.[10] The Vias de la Salud Health Promoter Program in Montgomery County, Maryland, used promotoras as trained lay volunteer health educators living in the Latino community. The promotoras conducted the training in schools, English-as-Second-Language adult classes, and in low-income housing facilities. After three years, a survey of parents indicated that 54 percent of the children increased their physical activity, 64 percent of the children increased their consumption of fresh fruits and vegetables, and 72 percent of the children were drinking water instead of sodas.

Community Level Planning and Evaluation

Planning for public health programs has two aspects: (1) the use of available and new resources in the best possible way, and (2) beginning the program when resources are sufficient to accomplish the goals. Of course, the environment (burden of disease, years of life lost due to premature death, and years lived with a disability) is important in the planning process.[11] In fact, before beginning a public health program, it must be decided whether the environment will allow the achievement of program objectives.

It is important to identify the objectives, the inputs, and the outcomes of a program. This must be done in the planning process before implementing the program. The planning process at the community level consists of identifying all stakeholders and gathering input from all involved. This information is a critical aspect of the program development because it is important to have as many stakeholders as possible engaged in the program and its future success.

Logic Models

A *logic model* is a graphic representation of the planning and implementation of a public health program. Logic models are used for both planning and evalua-

FIGURE 11.1: Basic logic model of resources, program activities, public health services, and expected changes in health

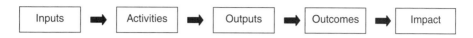

tion. The logic model is a tool that has been used for more than twenty years in public health. The benefit of using logic models is that they require the listing and inventory of available resources; planned program activities; the expected outputs; and short, intermediate, and long-term outcomes. The logic model graphically depicts the relationship between all of the components of the program.[12] Figure 11.1 shows a basic logic model. The model consists of inputs (resources, funding), activities (planned program activities that are implemented to achieve program objectives), outputs (public health services), outcomes (resulting changes in health or health behaviors), and impact of the program on the community.

An example of a logic model is shown in Figure 11.2. This model depicts the components of a family/school partnership program which focuses on a parent engagement. The logic model was developed to serve as a framework for program evaluation. The family involvement project is a national program focused on improving outcomes for children by increasing family member involvement (with a primary focus on parents).[13]

The basic components of a logic model are resources (called inputs), program activities, outputs, and outcomes. Inputs are human, financial, managerial, and community resources that are available for the planned program. Program activities are the processes, events, and actions that the program will implement to achieve its objectives, which usually involve a health change. Outputs, outcomes, and impact are the intended results of the program. Outputs are the direct results of the program activities, which may be public health services. Outcomes are the health changes that achieve the program's objectives. Outcomes can be short or long term. Short-term outcomes are expected to be seen in one to three years after the program has been implemented whereas long-term outcomes are expected to be achieved in four to six years. The impact is the health change that occurs as a result of the program. The impact is usually seen seven to ten years after the program has begun.

Logic models show the sequence of cause-and-effect relationships, which is a systems approach from the objectives to the program outcomes. Logic models connect the public health problem to the planned program (through the descrip-

FIGURE 11.2: Logic model for program evaluation

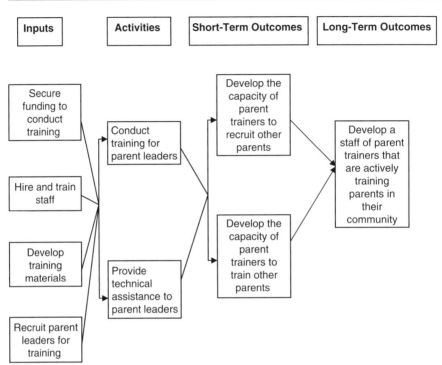

Source: Coffman J. Learning from logic models: An example of a family/school partnership. Harvard Family Research Project, 1999. http://www.hfrp.org/ publications-resources/publications-series/reaching-results/learning-from -logic-models-an-example-of-a-family-school-partnership-program.

tion of inputs and outputs) and the effects on the problem (described by the model outcome). If properly done, a logic model can be used to explain what aspects of the program achieved the objectives and how this achievement was accomplished.[14]

Logic models are also useful in identifying performance measurements that can be helpful in program evaluation. Perhaps the best benefit of a logic model is in planning and evaluation. It can be used for clear communication of the objectives of the program, the parts of the program, expected outcomes, and the impact of these outcomes. Many agree that given that all the parts of the program are depicted and specified, the logic model may best be used as an evaluation tool.[15,16]

Example of the Evaluation Process

Before discussing an example of the evaluation process, a few definitions will be presented. *Evaluation* has been defined as the collection and analysis of information to determine the relevance, progress, efficiency, effectiveness, and impact of a public health program.[17] *Relevance* indicates whether or not the program is needed. Progress indicates whether the program is being implemented, especially its activities, as planned. Efficiency is concerned with whether the program outcomes cost are reasonable or if the costs can be lowered to achieve the same outcomes. Effectiveness is concerned with whether the program achieves the planned objectives. Effectiveness evaluation focuses on program outputs. Impact is concerned with the long-term outcomes of the program. The evaluation of program impact is directed at determining whether the program outputs resulted in the planned effects on public health.

Two types of evaluations are summative and formative. *Summative evaluation* looks at the program activities and outcomes with respect to long-term effects. It determines whether the program has made an impact on the predetermined performance measurements. Types of summative evaluation include outcome evaluation, impact evaluation, cost-effectiveness and cost-benefit analyses, and meta-analysis. The summative evaluation process addresses what type of evaluation is adequate for the appropriate review of the program. In addition, it determines the effectiveness of the program, usually by using an observational method. The most important aspect is evaluating the impact of the program. This is usually done using cost-effectiveness and cost-benefit analyses, which indicate the net health benefit of the program for every dollar spent.

Formative evaluation reviews the activities that are part of the day-to-day operation of the program and is used to improve and manage the program. Types of formative evaluation include needs assessment, implementation evaluation, and process evaluation.[18] In formative evaluation, the core health problem is identified and defined by using focus groups of people in the community and other methods to get stakeholder input. Typically a needs assessment is conducted to determine the nature and seriousness of the health problem. Formative evaluation looks at possible ways to deliver the services and activities of the public health program. Decision analytical techniques are used to decide on the mode of delivery.

The evaluation of a school-based teenaged pregnancy program is an example of how a logic model can be both a planning and an evaluation tool. Teenaged pregnancy presents unique challenges to school nurses and teachers. A logic model was used to develop, implement, and evaluate a teenaged pregnancy program. The logic model served as a graphic depiction of program goals, activities, and outcomes. A communication method was used to explain the components of the program to all stakeholders. Because of the logic model's clearly focused structure, the success of the program was easily monitored.[19]

Examples

Many examples of community public health programming exist. The first involves participation at an urban senior citizen center.[20] An outreach program was developed that was intended to increase participation of a diverse group of low-income senior citizens. The senior center provided programs in health and wellness and other education. In addition, the senior citizens were able to get engaged in classes and group activities.

Community support for public health programming is often a critical aspect for success. In fact, community support may be one of many factors that affect public health programming. The University of Albany Prevention Research Center is using a community-based walking program to increase social support for physical activity.[21] Because increasing physical activity is affected by many factors, this program is partnering with communities to increase physical activity in rural areas. Before beginning the program, a community-based project was initiated to increase social support for physical activity. This project consisted of two rural communities testing the training materials and the physical activity program, which focused on walking in public buildings and existing fitness and walking trails.

Workplace health is an example of public health programming. It is known that workplace health promotion has a positive influence on the reduction of health risks. Workplace wellness programs have been implemented for several years and have proved successful.[22] One program is the New York City Department of Health and Mental Hygiene's Wellness at Work Program, which operates at twenty-seven work sites. This program focuses on health risk factors (for example, poor nutrition and smoking), weight-associated factors (for example, BMI and physical activity), and financial outcomes (health care utilization and absenteeism). The results of this program over a two-year period (2005 to 2007) indicate a slight decrease in health risk factors and financial savings at all sites. It is expected that greatest improvements will be seen as the program continues.

Drug use prevention is an urgent community concern. Many public health programs have been established, especially for school-aged children and adolescents. The Project ALERT program was instituted in middle schools in South Dakota. The purpose of the program is to reduce adolescents' use of illicit drugs. Project ALERT consisted of an educational curriculum taught in the middle schools. After eighteen months, the results of the program were evaluated. Project ALERT proved to be successful, with a 19 to 39 percent reduction in cigarette and marijuana use. The program was most effective in reducing the number of adolescents who start illicit drug use. As a side benefit, alcohol usage also declined.[23] This is an example of a public health program that is school based but has communitywide impact.

Public Health Programs

Public health planning and programming often occur at a national or regional geographical level. A prime example is the initiative known as Healthy People 2010.[24] This initiative was begun in January 2000 by the U.S. Department of Health and Human Services as a national health promotion and disease prevention program. The two major objectives of the program are to increase the quality and quantity, in years, of healthy life and to eliminate health disparities. Specifically, Healthy People 2010 presents objectives that are used to set a baseline for improving the health of Americans from 2000 to 2010. It is the third initiative of its kind to be used in the United States over the past thirty years.

NATIONAL CENTER FOR HEALTH STATISTICS (NCHS)

The NCHS is a part of the Centers for Disease Control and Prevention. The NCHS's principal role is as a health statistics agency. It compiles statistical information that is used to improve the health of people in the United States. The NCHS conducts periodic surveys, including the National Ambulatory Medical Care Survey, National Ambulatory Medical Care Survey, National Survey of Ambulatory Surgery, National Hospital Discharge Survey, National Nursing Home Survey, National Home and Hospice Care Survey, and National Survey of Residential Care Facilities.

Source: Centers for Disease Control and Prevention, http://www.cdc.gov/nchs.

Healthy People 2010 consists of 467 objectives that are divided into 28 focus areas. The target value for each objective is intended to be reached by 2010. In addition, a subset of the objectives has been identified as leading health indicators, selected because of available data to measure progress and their national interest. The leading health indicators are physical activity, overweight and obesity, tobacco use, substance abuse, responsible sexual behavior, mental health, injury and violence, environmental quality, immunization, and access to health care.

The progress of Healthy People 2010 is monitored by the National Center for Health Statistics (NCHS). The NCHS uses data that it collects, as well as information from more than 190 other sources, including private nongovernmental agencies. The NCHS evaluates the progress periodically and has a full midcourse review of the first five years. The evaluation looks at each objective and indicates whether the target has been met, the objective is improving, the objective is getting worse, there is little or no change, there is mixed progress, or the information is to be used to establish a baseline value for new objectives.

Figure 11.3 presents the 28 focus areas of Healthy People 2010. The 467 objectives are subdivided among these focus areas. Figure 11.4 shows information from the midcourse review of the progress of Healthy People 2010 for Objective 1–1, which is the first objective in the first focus area, access to quality health care services. Objective 1–1 states that 100 percent of people younger than 65 years will have health insurance by 2010. Figure 11.4 shows progress of this objective with respect to race and ethnic group. It is obvious that this target value of 100 percent has not been met by any of the groups depicted in the figure. However, progress can be seen in several groups since 1999. The only groups that have not experienced progress are whites and Hispanics, which remain the same. The greatest progress is seen in Native Hawaiians and Pacific Islanders.

Table 11.1 shows the objectives and target values in the focus area concerned with diabetes. There are seventeen objectives in the diabetes focus area, with fifteen currently active. Two objectives, 5–8 and 5–9, were eliminated during the midcourse review. The objectives cover education, incidence rate, prevalence rate, mortality rates, diagnostic testing, aspirin therapy, and self blood glucose monitoring. The objectives have different directions of achievement, depending on the intent of each. For example, objective 5–1 (diabetes education for people older than eighteen years) has a target of 60 percent, which is higher than what existed in 2000. The target value for objective 5–2 (three-year average of new cases of diabetes among people eighteen to eighty-four years of age) is 3.8 per 1,000 people in the population, which is lower than the average in 2000. In other words, the target values for good outcomes are higher than in 2000, and the target values for bad outcomes are lower.

The specific numerical value of the target value of each objective is related to its feasibility and the severity of the health outcome. For example, the target

FIGURE 11.3: Healthy People 2010 twenty-eight focus areas

Access to Quality Health Services

Arthritis, Osteoporosis and Chronic Back Conditions

Cancer

Chronic Kidney Disease

Diabetes

Disability and Secondary Conditions

Educational and Community-Based Programs

Environmental Health

Family Planning

Food Safety

Health Communication

Heart Disease and Stroke

HIV

Immunizations and Infectious Diseases

Injury and Violence Prevention

Maternal, Infant, and Child Health

Medical Product Safety

Mental Health and Mental Disorders

Nutrition and Overweight

Occupational Safety and Health

Oral Health

Physical Activity and Fitness

Public Health Infrastructure

Respiratory Diseases

Sexually Transmitted Diseases

Substance Abuse

Tobacco Use

Vision and Hearing

Source: Centers for Disease Control and Prevention, 2008.

FIGURE 11.4: Progress of objective 1–1

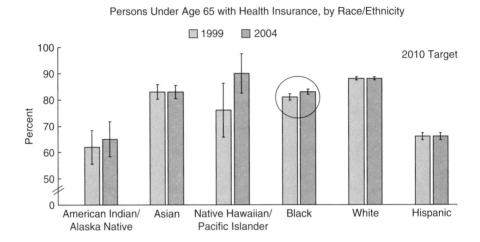

Persons Under Age 65 with Health Insurance, by Race/Ethnicity

I = 95% confidence interval.
Note: The black and white categories exclude persons of Hispanic origin. Persons of Hispanic origin may be any race. Respondents were asked to select one or more races. Data for the single race categories are for persons who reported only one racial group.

Obj. 1-1

Source: Centers for Disease Control, National Center for Health Statistics, http:www.cdc.gov/nchs/hphome.htm, 2008.

value for objective 5–17 (self blood glucose monitoring among people with diabetes, at least once a day among people eighteen years of age and older) is 61 percent. Ideally, you would hope that 100 percent of people with diabetes monitored their blood glucose levels. However, given the necessary education, patient compliance, and the needed testing equipment, 61 percent is a reasonable target value. The target value for objective 5–14 (annual foot examinations among people with diabetes who are eighteen years of age and older) is 91 percent. This target value is high because of the severity and resulting disability that is associated with lower extremity amputations. The higher percentage of people with diabetes who receive annual foot examinations is expected to result in a decrease in lower extremity amputations, less disability, and a higher quality of life.

Another example of public health planning at the national or regional level is Rural Healthy People 2010.[25] This plan was developed to study the application of Healthy People 2010 objectives for rural areas. This plan was the result of research literature and information gathering from rural communities and

TABLE 11.1: Diabetes Focus Area

Objective	Target Value
5–1 Diabetes education (18 years of age and older)	60%
5–2 New cases of diabetes, 3-year average (18 to 84 years of age)	3.8 per 1,000
5–3 Prevalence rate of diabetes	25 per 1,000
5–4 Proportion of people with diagnosed diabetes (20 years of age and older)	78%
5–5 Diabetes-related deaths	46 per 100,000
5–6 Diabetes-related deaths among people with diabetes	7.8 per 1,000
5–7 Cardiovascular disease deaths among people with diabetes	299 per 100,000
5–10 Lower extremity amputations among people with diabetes, 3-year average	2.9 per 1,000
5–11 Annual urinary microalbumin measurement among people with diabetes	14%
5–12 A_{1c} test at least twice a year among people with diabetes (18 years of age and older)	65%
5–13 Annual dilated eye examinations among people with diabetes (18 years of age and older)	76%
5–14 Annual foot examinations among people with diabetes (18 years of age and older)	91%
5–15 Annual dental examination among people with diabetes (2 years of age and older)	71%
5–16 Aspirin therapy among people with diabetes, at least 15 times a month (40 years of age and older)	30%
5–17 Self blood glucose monitoring among people with diabetes, at least once a day (18 years of age and older)	61%

Source: Centers for Disease Control and Prevention, 2008.

experts. Rural Healthy People 2010 is concerned with fifteen focus areas of the Healthy People 2010 that were identified as having importance to rural areas. The plan contains literature reviews and models for practice that link to the rural focus areas.

Figure 11.5 presents the Rural Healthy People 2010 selected focus areas. These areas were selected by using several methods, including roundtable discussions with rural health experts. The selection process was based on the following criteria: identification by rural experts as a high priority, overall prevalence rate in rural areas, disproportionate prevalence rate in rural areas, impact on mortality, contributor to other health problems, feasible solutions for rural areas, and known effective community interventions. The fifteen focus areas are listed in Figure 11.5 in their order of importance to rural health.

FIGURE 11.5: Rural Healthy People 2010 focus areas

Access to Quality Health Care Services

Mental Health

Oral Health

Educational and Community-based Programs

Diabetes

Injury and Violence Prevention

Nutrition and Overweight

Public Health Infrastructure

Tobacco Use

Maternal, Infant, and Child Health

Occupational Safety and Health

Cancer

Environmental Health

Heart Disease and Stroke

Source: Rural Healthy People 2010: A Companion Document for Rural Areas, Southwest Rural Health Research Center, School of Rural Public Health, The Texas A&M University System Health Science Center.

Public Health Agencies

The structure of the public health system is unique in the United States. The U.S. public health system consists of many types of governmental and nongovernmental agencies. These include over 3,000 county and city health departments and local boards of health. In addition, there are 59 state and territorial health departments as well as tribal health departments. Supporting this system are more than 160,000 public and private laboratories and hospitals and volunteer organizations such as the Red Cross. The public health system in the United States is a combination of federal, state, and local health agencies.[26]

In general, public health organizations provide epidemiological investigations of diseases, laboratory testing, health promotion, health education, and information gathering, analysis, interpretation, and dissemination. Federal, state, and local laws govern public health. Federal influence comes in the form of funding and issues of interstate commerce. However, most public health authority (for example, disease reporting, health care provider and facility licensing) belongs to the states.[27] The states usually exercise this authority as police power to protect the public's health, enforcing safety and sanitary codes, conducting inspections, reporting notifiable diseases, and licensing health care providers and facilities.[28]

The organizational structure of state health departments is also unique. More than twenty-five states have a centralized, stand-alone structure. The remaining state health departments are decentralized, with the local health agencies conducting public health services. In about 25 percent of the states, there is a shared organizational relationship, with the state agency supporting local agencies as needed.[29] The majority of state health departments have a governing board, with members from the community, the health care industry, and government. Almost all state health agencies are led by a state health officer. The governor typically appoints the state health officer.

Summary

Community health is synonymous with public health, and it is concerned with the health of the people in a community. A community can be a small number of people or a large population. A community can be defined by a location that is common to a number of people. Community health programs have been undertaken to improve the health of populations. Healthy People 2010 is one such program that established objectives for the health of a community. Community health workers are people who work in the community to improve health.

It is important to evaluate community health programs because of their cost and impact on a large number of people. Logic models represent one way to evaluate programs. Program evaluation is needed to decide whether to continue, expand, or stop program efforts.

Key Terms

Community, 212

Community health workers, 213

Evaluation, 217

Formative evaluation, 217

Healthy People 2010, 219

Joint actions, 212

Location, 212

Logic model, 214

Relevance, 217

Sharing, 212

Social connections, 212

Summative evaluation, 217

Chapter Exercises

1. Define the term *community* and discuss how it affects health.
2. Discuss the effects of social connections on communities.
3. Describe the different structures of state health agencies in the United States.
4. Define what is meant by a community health worker.
5. What is an important characteristic of community health workers?

Chapter Review

1. The leading health indicators in Healthy People 2010 include
   a. physical activity.
   b. overweight and obesity.
   c. tobacco use.
   d. immunization.
   e. access to health care.
   f. all of the above.
2. Sharing refers to common interests and perceptions of the people who contribute to the feeling of community. True or False?
3. The main objectives of Healthy People 2010 are
   a. cost containment and access to care.
   b. quantity and quality of a healthy life and elimination of health disparities.
   c. cost containment and quality of life.
   d. all of the above.
   e. none of the above.
4. Most state departments of health have a centralized organizational structure. True or False?
5. Logic models
   a. are useful for planning only.
   b. are useful for evaluation only.
   c. show the sequence of cause-and-effect relationships.
   d. none of the above.
6. Types of summative evaluation include
   a. outcome evaluation.
   b. cost-effectiveness.
   c. cost-benefit analyses.
   d. all of the above.
   e. none of the above.

7. Types of formative evaluation include
    a. outcome evaluation.
    b. cost-effectiveness.
    c. cost-benefit analyses.
    d. needs assessment.
    e. all of the above.
    f. none of the above.

Answer True or False for the following statements.

8. A key to success for community health workers is that they live in the communities in which they work.

9. Unlike other community health workers, promotoras do not live in their communities, but are successful because they all speak Spanish fluently.

10. One of the aspects of planning for public health programs is the use of available and new resources in the best possible way.

EPIDEMIOLOGY TODAY

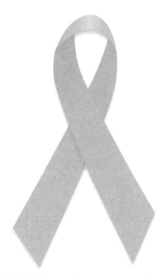

Emergency Preparedness

Surveillance

The events of September 11, 2001, changed the United States forever in many ways. The result has been an increase in military and civil awareness and a change in the manner in which public health is viewed by the people in the United States. Public health agencies will continue to provide health services as usual, but they are now also expected to be prepared for terrorism events.

Terrorism preparedness and response planning use epidemiology. Public health surveillance and epidemiological response plans for terrorism events are the centerpieces of any local, regional, state, or national system. Public health activities include using disease surveillance as a part of terrorism response planning. Surveillance teams are used to conduct epidemiological investigations of suspected or confirmed biological or chemical terrorism events. These surveillance programs include specific diseases (for example, influenza and anthrax) and syndromic diseases (a group of symptoms that collectively indicate or characterize a disease, psychological disorder, or other abnormal condition). A well-known syndromic disease is AIDS.[1]

In May 2003, it was estimated that a syndromic surveillance system had been implemented at more than one hundred locations in the United States. Syndromic surveillance systems are intended to monitor disease syndromes that may be indicative of a bioterrorism *disease*. These surveillance systems are focused on the early detection of bioterrorism-related epidemics. The theory of syndromic surveillance is that during an attack or a disease outbreak, people who are affected will become ill and be absent from work or school. After a short time, they will seek treatment from a physician. Syndromic surveillance systems must include monitoring of works and school absenteeism, the use of over-the-counter medications, and visits to hospitals and physicians.[2]

Syndromic surveillance systems have been established that target the following bioterrorism-related diseases: inhalational anthrax, tularemia, pneumonic plague, botulism, smallpox, and viral hemorrhagic fevers.[3] New diseases are added to the notifiable disease surveillance systems; examples include diseases caused by variola, *Francisella tularensis,* and *Brucella melitensis.*

SYNDROMIC SURVEILLANCE

Syndromic surveillance uses health-related information that indicates a strong probability of a case or an outbreak that would result in a public health response. Syndromic surveillance is used for detecting outbreaks associated with bioterrorism and is increasingly being explored by public health officials. Diseases that are under syndromic surveillance are anthrax, botulism, plague, smallpox, tularemia, and viral hemorrhagic fever.

Source: Centers for Disease Control and Prevention, http://www.cdc.gov/ncphi/disss/nndss/syndromic.htm.

Planning

Terrorism before September 11, 2001, was something that happened in other parts of the world and, as it was then thought, could never occur in the United States. Public health agencies have been concerned with the possibility of terrorism for many years, but the events of September 11 have caused a heightened level of alert. The challenge for public health is that terrorism preparedness planning requires cooperation and coordination with new partners. For the first time, public health agencies are working closely with the Federal Bureau of Investigation, state emergency management agencies, local fire and police authorities, the U.S. Department of Justice, and the U.S. Department of Defense.

This new level of concern and the necessity of working with new and additional partners have resulted in a more formal planning process. Public health agencies need to sustain and strengthen these relationships. Public health agencies must not lose focus on the health component of planning, and they must identify and work with partners who can assist in achieving planning objectives.[4]

The remainder of this chapter focuses on global health and the infectious and chronic diseases that are important today. The attention to emergency preparedness and global health may be the most important concern for public health and epidemiology now and into the near future. Emergency preparedness, global health, and infectious and chronic diseases are related aspects of public health today.

Global Health

Global health is the health of populations in the world; it exceeds the health concerns of individual nations. Global health organizations such as WHO seek to improve worldwide health and protect populations against health threats that cross national borders. Both infectious and chronic diseases threaten global health.

Infectious Diseases

HIV/AIDS

HIV is transmitted in many ways: by unprotected sexual intercourse, oral sex with an HIV-infected person, transfusion of contaminated blood, and the sharing of contaminated needles and syringes. There is also the possibility of HIV transmission between a pregnant mother and her infant child.

It is not known exactly how long it takes for a person who is HIV-infected to develop AIDS, but it is known that most HIV-infected people who do not receive treatment will have clinical signs between five and ten years after infection. The time between HIV infection and the development of AIDS can take between ten and fifteen years. The major clinical manifestation of HIV/AIDS is TB. In fact, TB is the leading cause of death in Africa in people who are HIV infected.

Table 12.1 presents information about HIV infection and deaths due to AIDS. Globally it has been estimated that more than 33 million people are living with HIV infection. Almost 31 million are adults, and 2 million are children. It has also been estimated that 2.7 million new cases of HIV infection occur each year, 2 million among adults and 370,000 among children. In 2007, 2 million people died of AIDS; 270,000 of those deaths were children.

Table 12.2 shows information about the number of people receiving treatment for HIV/AIDS in the world. About two thirds of the people receiving treatment live in sub-Saharan Africa: 22 million of the total 33 million. More

TABLE 12.1: Global Summary of AIDS Epidemic, December 2007

	Total	Adults	Children Younger Than 15 Years
People living with HIV	33,000,000	30,800,000	2,000,000
People newly infected with HIV in 2007	2,700,000	2,000,000	370,000
AIDS deaths in 2007	2,000,000	1,800,000	270,000

Source: World Health Organization, 2008: http://www.unaids.org/en/KnowledgeCentre/ HIVData/EpiUpdate/EpiUpdArchive/2007/default.asp.

TABLE 12.2: Estimated Number of People Receiving Antiretroviral Therapy by Region, December 2003 to December 2007

Area	Adults and Children Living with HIV	Adults and Children Newly Infected with HIV	Adult Prevalence Rate, %	Adult and Child Deaths Due to AIDS
Sub-Saharan Africa	22,000,000	1,900,000	5.0	1,500,000
Middle East and North Africa	380,000	40,000	0.3	27,000
South and Southeast Asia	4,200,000	330,000	0.3	340,000
East Asia	740,000	52,000	0.1	40,000
Latin America	1,700,000	140,000	0.5	63,000
Caribbean	230,000	20,000	1.1	14,000
Eastern Europe and Central Asia	1,500,000	110,000	0.8	58,000
Western and Central Europe	730,000	27,000	0.3	8,000
North America	1,200,000	13,000	0.4	23,000
Oceania	74,000	13,000	0.4	1,000
Total	32,754,000	2,645,000	0.8	2,074,000

Source: World Health Organization.

than half of newly infected cases of HIV infection are also seen in sub-Saharan Africa. The adult prevalence rate is 5.0 percent in sub-Saharan Africa, the highest in all regions of the world. Adults and children who died of AIDS equaled 2 million, with 1.5 million deaths in sub-Saharan Africa.

By the end of 2007, more than 3 million people in low-income countries were receiving treatment for HIV infection. This number has increased over the past few years because HIV drugs have become more available. There is no known cure for HIV infection, but if a person receives treatment medications, the progression to AIDS can be significantly slowed.[5]

Bird Flu

Bird flu, also called *avian influenza,* is an infectious disease seen in birds. Bird flu is caused by type A strains of the influenza virus. The effect of the infection in birds ranges from a mild illness to a quickly developing deadly disease. It is unusual to find avian influenza virus in humans, but cases of severe respiratory disease have occurred in humans. Those who have become infected usually had close contact with infected birds (especially chickens).

The main fear about bird flu is the possibility of a pandemic epidemic in humans. The last influenza pandemic happened in 1968. A strain of avian influenza, H5N1, has infected humans, but no person-to-person transmission has occurred. Again, the fear is mutation of the strain until it gets transmitted person-to-person, resulting in an outbreak of pandemic proportions. Because of the ability of the H5N1 virus to change, prevention and medical treatments could become ineffective. WHO has established a plan to address the fear of a pandemic. This plan includes reducing human exposure to the H5N1 virus, enhancing the global early warning systems, increasing the ability of countries to respond to a pandemic, and promoting research and development of vaccines and antiviral medications. WHO established the Global Influenza Program to coordinate activities of the plan.

Table 12.3 presents the cumulative number of confirmed human cases of avian influenza from 2003 to 2008. The largest number of cases were seen in Indonesia, closely followed by Vietnam. The number of cases peaked across the world during 2005 and 2007 and significantly decreased in 2008. For example, in Thailand, twenty-five cases have occurred from 2003 to 2008, but there have been no cases since 2006.

Table 12.4 shows the cumulative number of confirmed human deaths from avian influenza from 2003 to 2008. The total number of deaths equaled 245, which represents 63.3 percent of cases. Again, Indonesia had the greatest number of deaths, and Vietnam had the second highest. Most deaths occurred between 2004 and 2007, with a significant decrease in 2008.

West Nile Virus

The West Nile virus has been causing severe disease in the United States since the late 1990s. The West Nile virus can cause West Nile encephalitis and West Nile meningitis, which are characterized by inflammation of the brain and the

TABLE 12.3: Cumulative Number of Confirmed Human Cases of
Avian Influenza A (H5N1), 2003 to 2008

Country	2003	2004	2005	2006	2007	2008	Total
Azerbaijan	0	0	0	8	0	0	8
Bangladesh	0	0	0	0	0	1	1
Cambodia	0	0	4	2	1	0	7
China	1	0	8	13	5	3	30
Djibouti	0	0	0	1	0	0	1
Egypt	0	0	0	18	25	7	50
Indonesia	0	0	20	55	42	20	137
Iraq	0	0	0	3	0	0	3
Lao People's Democratic Republic	0	0	0	0	2	0	2
Myanmar	0	0	0	1	0	0	1
Nigeria	0	0	0	0	1	0	1
Pakistan	0	0	0	0	3	0	3
Thailand	0	17	5	3	0	0	25
Turkey	0	0	0	12	0	0	12
Vietnam	3	29	61	0	8	5	106
Total	4	46	98	115	88	36	387

Source: World Health Organization, http://www.who.int/csr/disease/avian_influenza/
country/cases_table_2008_09_10/en/index.html.

TABLE 12.4: Cumulative Number of Confirmed Human Deaths
from Avian Influenza A (H5N1), 2003 to 2008

Country	2003	2004	2005	2006	2007	2008	Total
Azerbaijan	0	0	0	5	0	0	5
Bangladesh	0	0	0	0	0	0	0
Cambodia	0	0	4	2	1	0	7
China	1	0	5	8	3	3	20
Djibouti	0	0	0	0	0	0	0
Egypt	0	0	0	10	9	3	22
Indonesia	0	0	13	45	37	17	112
Iraq	0	0	0	2	0	0	2
Lao People's Democratic Republic	0	0	0	0	2	0	2
Myanmar	0	0	0	0	0	0	0
Nigeria	0	0	0	0	1	0	1
Pakistan	0	0	0	0	1	0	1
Thailand	0	12	2	3	0	0	17
Turkey	0	0	0	4	0	0	4
Vietnam	3	20	19	0	5	5	52
Total	4	32	43	79	59	28	245

Source: World Health Organization: http://www.who.int/csr/disease/avian_influenza/
country/cases_table_2008_09_10/en/index.html.

membrane around the brain and the spinal cord. It also causes a less severe condition called West Nile fever, which is a reportable disease that does not appear to cause neurological problems.

Table 12.5 presents information about the amount of disease that has been caused by West Nile virus in 2008. Of the total number of cases reported, 46 percent consisted of West Nile meningitis or encephalitis. Slightly more than half (51 percent) of the cases were West Nile fever. The remaining cases are unspecified.

It is important to remember that severe cases are more likely to be reported, so in reality the proportion of severe cases is probably much lower than 46 percent. This is the result of disease reporting bias. In fact, some population surveys have shown that the proportion of severe cases is less than 10 percent.[6]

Methicillin-Resistant Staphylococcus aureus

Methicillin-resistant Staphylococcus aureus (MRSA) is a potentially severe type of staph bacteria that is resistant to some antibiotics. MRSA typically causes skin and other infections. It is usually transmitted by direct contact with an infected person, especially by sharing clothing, towels, and the like. Skin infections appear as bumps or infected areas that are usually red, swollen, and painful. The areas may have pus or other fluid drainage. These skin infections are usually seen in people who also have a fever.[7]

The spread of MRSA usually happens in places where people are in close contact, including schools and locker rooms, where students and athletes often share personal items. MRSA may be spread by touching infected areas or contaminated items. These items may be contaminated by direct contact with infected areas or by contaminated hands, spreading the bacteria.

MRSA can be prevented by keeping surfaces free of bacteria. This includes covering infected areas with bandages and changing these bandages often. Another prevention tactic is to frequently wash and clean your hands, especially after changing bandages. Areas must be kept clean, including furniture (such as benches in a locker room) and table tops.[8]

Emerging Diseases

The CDC has identified several emerging infectious diseases. These are diseases that have been infrequently seen in the population until recently or diseases that have been occurring in other parts of the world with a potential to spread. Table

TABLE 12.5: West Nile Virus Activity, United States, 2008

State	Encephalitis or Meningitis	Fever	Other	Total Cases	Deaths
Alabama	10	9	0	19	0
Arizona	47	24	6	77	3
Arkansas	8	0	0	8	0
California	211	110	8	329	7
Colorado	13	64	0	77	0
Connecticut	4	2	1	7	0
Delaware	0	0	1	1	0
Florida	2	0	0	2	0
Georgia	3	3	1	7	0
Idaho	1	29	2	32	0
Illinois	11	4	4	19	1
Indiana	2	0	1	3	0
Iowa	5	1	3	9	1
Kansas	5	20	0	25	0
Kentucky	2	0	1	3	0
Louisiana	9	27	0	36	0
Maryland	7	5	1	13	0
Michigan	7	4	3	14	0
Minnesota	3	18	0	21	0
Mississippi	31	65	1	97	3
Missouri	9	7	0	16	1
Montana	0	3	2	5	0
Nebraska	4	33	0	37	0
Nevada	8	5	2	15	0
New Jersey	3	4	0	7	1
New Mexico	3	1	0	4	0
New York	28	11	0	29	6
North Dakota	2	41	0	43	0
Ohio	14	1	1	16	1
Oklahoma	3	5	0	8	0
Oregon	0	4	0	4	0
Pennsylvania	5	0	0	5	0
Rhode Island	1	0	0	1	0
South Dakota	11	28	0	39	0
Tennessee	5	6	0	11	0
Totals	486	534	5	1,025	24

Source: Centers for Disease Control and Prevention, Center for Vector-Borne Infectious Diseases, 2008.

TABLE 12.6: Emerging Infectious Diseases

Drug-resistant infections	Hendra virus infection	Pertussis
Bovine spongiform encephalopathy (mad cow disease) and variant Creutzfeldt-Jakob disease	Histoplasmosis	Plague
	HIV/AIDS	Poliomyelitis
	Influenza	Rabies
	Lassa fever	Rift Valley fever
Campylobacteriosis	Legionnaires' disease and Pontiac fever	Rotavirus infection
Chagas' disease		Salmonellosis
Cholera	Leptospirosis	Severe acute respiratory syndrome (SARS)
Cryptococcosis	Listeriosis	
Cryptosporidiosis	Lyme disease	Shigellosis
Cyclosporiasis	Malaria	Smallpox
Cysticercosis	Marburg hemorrhagic fever	Sleeping sickness
Dengue fever		Tuberculosis
Diphtheria	Measles	Tularemia
Ebola hemorrhagic fever	Meningitis	Valley fever
Escherichia coli infection	Monkeypox	Vancomycin-intermediate/resistant *Staphylococcus aureus* (VISA/VRSA)
Group B streptococcal infection	Methicillin-resistant *Staphylococcus aureus* (MRSA)	
Hantavirus pulmonary syndrome	Nipah virus infection	West Nile virus infection
Hepatitis C	Norovirus infection	Yellow fever

Source: Centers for Disease Control and Prevention, http://www.cdc.gov/ncidod/diseases/eid/index.htm.

12.6 shows the list of emerging infectious diseases, including mad cow disease, Lyme disease, tularemia, SARS, MRSA, Legionnaires' disease, and H1N1 flu.

Mad Cow Disease

Mad cow disease, also called *bovine spongiform encephalopathy,* is a progressive neurological disorder seen in cattle. The infectious agent is a prion, which is a modified form of a protein. The modification results in a harmful agent that attacks the central nervous system of cattle. Mad cow disease was first seen in the United Kingdom.[9]

The mad cow disease epidemic began in the 1980s when cattle were fed infected feed. The infected feed was used throughout the United Kingdom and resulted in about 1,000 new cases each week during January 1993. The first human cases were reported in the United Kingdom in 1996. The human form of mad cow disease is called variant. Creutzfeldt-Jakob disease. In response to the epidemic, all animals older than thirty months were removed from human use, which has been effective.

Since the first cases were identified in the United Kingdom, eighteen cases of mad cow disease in cattle have been seen in North America: three in the United States and fifteen in Canada. Since 2006 all cases of mad cow disease in cattle have been found in Canada.[10]

Cholera

Cholera is caused by the bacterium *Vibrio cholerae*, and it affects humans in the form of an acute, diarrheal disease that has varying symptoms. About 5 percent of people infected will have vomiting, leg cramps, and watery diarrhea. These people may experience dehydration and shock, and those who do not receive treatment can die in a matter of hours. Because cholera can be easily treated and prevented, it is not a major public health concern.[11]

Cholera is rare in developed countries, but it is common in the Indian sub-continent and sub-Saharan Africa. In 1991 a cholera epidemic was identified in South America that quickly became a pandemic. In the United States, cholera does not usually occur because of modern sewage and water treatment systems. The concern with this disease is that with improved transportation and increased travel to other countries, especially Africa, Asia, and Latin America, more people from the United States may be exposed to the bacteria.[12]

Ebola Hemorrhagic Fever

Ebola hemorrhagic fever, which is caused by infection from the Ebola virus, was first seen in 1976. It is a severe disease in humans and primates (monkeys, gorillas, and chimpanzees) that can result in death. It is named after a river in the Democratic Republic of the Congo and is caused by an RNA virus.

It is thought that Ebola virus is a zoonotic (animal-borne) infectious agent that normally exists in animal hosts native to Africa. The virus is not thought to be native to other parts of the world, but these animal hosts may be transported around the world. Despite what researchers think, there is not a known natural reservoir of the Ebola virus.[13]

Cases of Ebola hemorrhagic fever have been seen in many parts of Africa. Ebola hemorrhagic fever cases usually are seen in sporadic outbreaks and often spread within a health care setting. It is likely that sporadic, isolated cases occur as well, but go unrecognized. No cases have been seen in the United States.

The first person to get infected in an Ebola epidemic probably would have had contact with an infected animal. This person can start an epidemic by infecting others from direct contact with blood or other body fluids. The epidemic can spread quickly because family and friends of the infected person come into close contact. Ebola hemorrhagic fever can spread in a health care facility (hospital or clinic) by nosocomial (infections resulting from treatment in a hospital or a health care facility) transmission.[14]

Escherichia coli Infection

Escherichia coli (known as *E. coli*) infections can cause several different symptoms, including diarrhea, urinary tract infections, respiratory problems, and pneumonia. Strains of *E. coli* are harmful because they produce a toxin called Shiga toxin. *E. coli* can affect all people, but the young and old are at highest risk.

The symptoms of infections caused by the Shiga toxin include diarrhea, stomach cramps, and vomiting. Fever may occur, but it will not be high. The infections may be mild or severe, but most people are better within a week. In a small proportion of infected people, hemolytic uremic syndrome will develop. This disease syndrome includes kidney failure and other serious problems. Recovery occurs in the majority of people, but some will suffer permanent damage or die.[15]

E. coli infections are spread by the consumption of contaminated food, unpasteurized milk, and contaminated water. Specific foods that are at high risk for *E. coli* include unpasteurized milk, unpasteurized apple cider, and cheeses made from unpasteurized milk. Infections can also be spread when food is consumed that was prepared by someone who does not wash their hands after using the toilet.

Group B Streptococcal Infection

Group B streptococcus causes illness in pregnant women, newborns, the elderly, and people with diabetes or liver disease. In fact, group B streptococcus is the major cause of life-threatening infections in newborns. These infections are sepsis (a blood infection) and meningitis. Group B streptococcus also causes pneumonia in newborns.[16]

Most infections in newborns will occur in the first week of life and usually result in sepsis, meningitis, and pneumonia. Premature babies are at a higher risk for group B streptococcal infections, but full-term babies mostly get sick. Meningitis is more often seen several months after birth.

Hepatitis C

Hepatitis C is a contagious liver disease caused by a virus. It is spread from the blood of an infected person to others through sharing needles or other items used to inject drugs. Hepatitis C can be a mild problem that lasts for weeks, or it can become a lifelong ailment.

Hepatitis C once was spread through blood transfusions and organ transplants, but since 1992, when universal precautions began, no cases have been reported. It can be spread through sexual intercourse, and the risk of infection increases if one has multiple sex partners. People who are HIV infected are at high risk for hepatitis C. Hepatitis C is not spread by breastfeeding, kissing, coughing, sneezing, or through food and water.

Legionnaires' Disease

Legionnaires' disease is a respiratory tract disease that has the same signs and symptoms as different types of pneumonia. It is caused by the *Legionella* species bacteria and is seen as a lung infection. The bacteria and disease got its name in 1976 after many people became ill, and some died, at an American Legion convention in Philadelphia. Today between 8,000 and 18,000 people are diagnosed with Legionnaires' disease in the United States each year.[17]

The symptoms of Legionnaires' disease begin about two days after exposure to the bacteria. A mild infection can result, known as Pontiac fever, that lasts two to five days. With the fever, people may have headaches and muscle aches but not pneumonia. If Legionnaires' disease develops into pneumonia, up to 30 percent of people may die. But most cases can be treated with antibiotics.

The *Legionella* bacteria are found in the environment and grow and multiply in warm water. Typically places that *Legionella* bacteria are found include hot tubs, cooling towers, hot water tanks, or air-conditioning systems in large buildings. People get infected by inhaling the bacteria that are in water mists or vapors. People who are at most risk for Legionnaires' disease are older individuals (age sixty-five and older) and people who smoke or have chronic lung disease. The disease is not spread from person to person. *Legionella* outbreaks are point-source epidemics in which several cases of a disease occur within a few days or hours due to exposure to a common source of infection such as food or water.[18]

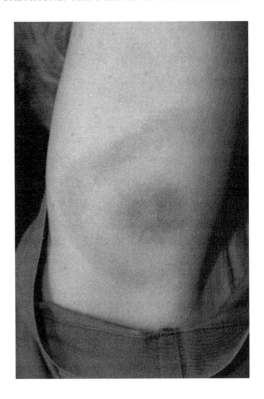

Lyme Disease

Lyme disease was first reported in the United States in the town of Old Lyme, Connecticut, in 1975. Cases have now been reported in most parts of the United States. Lyme disease is transmitted to humans through ticks. Infected ticks bite humans and transmit the bacterium *Borrelia burgdorferi*. Infected people are typically fatigued and have fever, headache, and a skin rash. Lyme disease cases are treated with antibiotics, with most people improving in a few weeks. If untreated, the infection can cause heart and nervous system problems.

Malaria

Malaria is a disease that is spread by indirect contact with a mosquito. People usually get malaria by being bitten by an infected female *Anopheles* mosquito. Malaria is caused by a parasite that lives in the mosquito and is characterized by fever, chills, and flulike symptoms. Four malaria parasites are capable of causing disease in humans. If malaria is not treated, the complications can lead to death. In fact, more than a million people die each year from malaria.

Malaria is most prevalent in sub-Saharan Africa. It is a concern for travelers to this part of the world, but a preventive drug can be taken. In the United States, more than a thousand cases are diagnosed each year. These cases mostly occur in travelers who have recently visited or are immigrants from areas of the world where malaria is prevalent.

Measles

Measles is a respiratory tract disease caused by a virus that causes a rash, high temperature, a cough, and watery eyes. Measles usually lasts about one week. The problem with measles is the complications that are associated with the condition, including diarrhea, ear infections, pneumonia, encephalitis, seizures, and even death.

Measles is transmitted directly from person to person through coughing and sneezing. It is highly contagious, and 90 percent of people who come in contact with an infected person will become infected. Measles can be transmitted four days before and four days after a skin rash appears. If someone is not immunized against measles, they will eventually get infected if exposed to the virus.

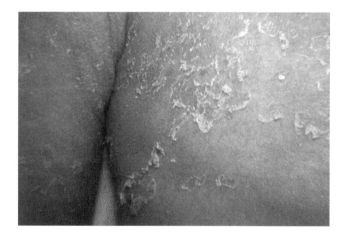

Poliomyelitis

Poliomyelitis is caused by a virus that attacks the nervous system. The vast majority of people who are infected have no symptoms. About 1 percent of infected people will develop permanent paralysis, usually of the legs. Death may occur when the paralysis moves to the respiratory system. Poliomyelitis is transmitted through contact with an infected person.

Poliomyelitis can be prevented by vaccination. It is important that children be vaccinated with four dosages, beginning at age two months and following with a booster between the ages of four and six years. Adults should be vaccinated if they are traveling to an area of the world where poliomyelitis is endemic.[19]

Salmonellosis

Salmonellosis is an infection caused by a *Salmonella* species bacterium known to cause illness in humans for the past one hundred years. The most common symptoms are fever, diarrhea, and abdominal cramps within twelve to seventy-two hours of infection. Salmonellosis lasts for four to seven days, with hospitalization needed if the diarrhea becomes severe.

Salmonella bacteria are transmitted to humans through food that is contaminated with animal feces. Typical foods are beef, poultry, milk, or eggs. Contaminated vegetables are not usually the source of the infection. Cooking foods destroys *Salmonella*, but the infection can be spread by the hands of infected food workers.[20]

SARS

SARS was first reported in Asia in 2003. It is a respiratory tract illness that is caused by a coronavirus. SARS causes a high temperature, followed by headaches and body aches. Within six months of its discovery, the SARS pandemic spread through countries in Asia, Europe, North America, and South America; more than 8,000 people were infected, with 774 deaths.[21]

Little is known about SARS and how the epidemic started or ended. It is known that SARS is spread through person-to-person contact, and it is thought that it is transmitted by respiratory droplets from coughing and sneezing. The infection can also be spread when people come into contact with the droplets on surfaces of furniture. It is suspected that SARS can be spread through the air or other unknown ways. Reducing your contact with someone with SARS lowers the risk for the disease. According to the CDC, hand hygiene is the most important aspect of SARS prevention. This might include hand washing or cleaning hands with an alcohol-based hand sanitizer.

Tuberculosis

In the past decade, TB has become a concern again after almost disappearing in the United States during the 1980s. It is caused by *Mycobacterium tuberculosis*, which attacks the lungs in humans. TB is potentially fatal and many years ago was the leading cause of death in the United States. TB spreads from person to person through the air when a person with the active disease coughs or sneezes.

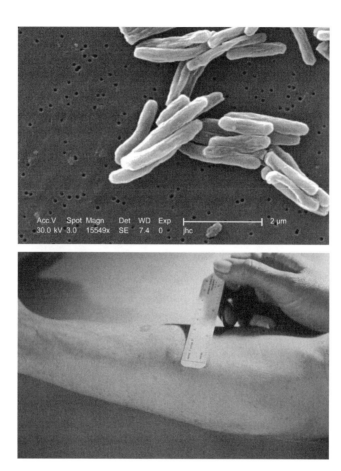

Some people who have been infected do not develop active TB or get sick. They have latent TB, which can develop into active TB if it is not treated. Because TB was once a major cause of death, medications have been developed that have significantly decreased the number of infected people. However, the disease has experienced a resurgence, and today more than 15,000 cases of TB are reported each year. This reappearance has been attributed to compromised immune systems in people with AIDS, diabetes mellitus, leukemia, kidney disease, and head or neck cancer.[22]

Tularemia

Tularemia is caused by the bacterium *Francisella tularensis*, which is found in rodents, rabbits, and hares in the United States. Tularemia causes fever, chills, diarrhea, muscle aches, joint pain, a dry cough, and body weakness. People with tularemia are at risk for the development of pneumonia. Tularemia also causes ulcers of the skin or mouth, swollen and painful lymph glands, swollen and painful eyes, and sore throat.

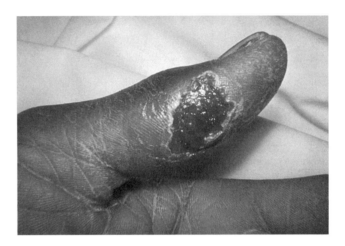

Tularemia is spread in several ways, including eating or drinking contaminated food or water, breathing in the bacteria, and bites from infected ticks or deerflies. It is not spread from person to person, so people with tularemia do not require isolation. Early treatment with antibiotics is important as tularemia may result in death if not properly treated. Because of its infectivity, tularemia has the potential to be used as a biological weapon. If the bacteria were made airborne, infection would occur quickly after inhaling. People who inhaled the bacteria would develop deadly pneumonia and systemic infection.[23]

H1N1 Flu

H1N1 flu is considered a new flu virus that was first seen in the United States in 2009. H1N1 flu is a global problem because it spreads from person to person. In fact, in June 2009 WHO stated that H1N1 flu was a pandemic.

The H1N1 influenza virus was thought to be a form of swine flu because laboratory testing showed that many of the genes in this new virus were similar to influenza viruses that normally occur in pigs (swine) in North America. But further study has shown that the H1N1 virus is different from what normally circulates in North American pigs and that it is actually a new flu virus. H1N1 flu is a contagious disease that spreads from human to human. One of the troubling characteristics of H1N1 flu is that it spreads year-round, not just during the traditional flu season.[24]

Chronic Diseases

As discussed in previous chapters, chronic diseases are the major concern for the health of people. The major chronic diseases and conditions are heart disease, diabetes, arthritis, obesity, breast cancer, colorectal cancer, cervical cancer, and asthma. These diseases and conditions are described below.

Heart Disease

Heart disease is the leading cause of death in the United States. The death rate from heart disease is highest in whites, followed closely by blacks.[25] Among all of the heart disease conditions, coronary heart disease is the most prevalent and accounts for the vast majority of deaths from heart disease.[26] Coronary heart disease kills more than 7 million people each year across the world.[27] Heart disease deaths usually occur before people can receive treatment.[28]

In 2005 more than 24 million people were diagnosed with heart disease. Of all the people older than eighteen years who were hospitalized in that year, 11 percent were admitted to receive treatment for heart disease.[29] In 2006, 4.2 million hospital discharges were attributed to heart disease, and the average length of stay in a hospital for people receiving treatment for heart disease was 4.4 days. With respect to mortality, 652,091 people died in 2005 from heart disease, which is a mortality rate of 222 deaths per 100,000 people in the population.[30]

Arthritis

Arthritis is a broad term that describes many diseases and conditions of the joints in the body and the tissues that surround the joints and connective tissue. These rheumatic diseases and conditions are characterized by stiffness and pain in the joints. About 46 million people have been diagnosed with some form of arthritis in the United States. Almost 10 percent of these people have limitations in movement and activity because of arthritis.[31] It is estimated that by 2030, a total of 67 million people older than eighteen years will have diagnosed arthritis. About 40 percent of these people will have activity limitations that can be attributed to arthritis.

Arthritis has been identified as the cause of more than 140,000 deaths during the past twenty years. Today almost 10,000 deaths occur each year that can be attributed to arthritis, with an annual mortality rate of 3 deaths per 100,000 people in the population. The mortality rate is higher in African Americans and in women. Three of the arthritis or rheumatic conditions cause 80 percent of deaths: systemic lupus erythematosus, vasculitis, and rheumatoid arthritis.[32]

Breast Cancer

Breast cancer is the second most common cancer to affect women. It is the leading cause of death in Hispanic women and the second most common cause in other women. Information from 2004 indicated that more than 185,000 women were diagnosed with breast cancer. In that same year, more than 40,000 women died of breast cancer. Many people do not know that men can also develop breast cancer. In 2004 more than 1,800 men were diagnosed with breast cancer, and over 360 died.[33]

There are two types of breast cancer, ductal and lobular carcinoma. Ductal carcinoma is the most prevalent and can occur in two ways. Ductal carcinoma in situ occurs in the cells that line the milk ducts and does not spread to other areas of the breast. Invasive ductal carcinoma starts in the milk ducts, then spreads into other parts of the breast and the body. Lobular carcinoma begins in the lobules of the breast. The lobules are the glands that produce milk. Lobular carcinoma has two forms, lobular carcinoma in situ and invasive lobular carcinoma. Cancer cells of lobular carcinoma in situ are found only in the lobules, but cancer cells of invasive lobular carcinoma can spread through the body.

Obesity

Obesity is excess body fat. It is linked to higher LDL (bad) cholesterol and triglyceride levels and to lower HDL (good) cholesterol, high blood pressure, and diabetes. The prevalence of obesity in the United States, which is defined as a

TABLE 12.7: Obesity Prevalence Rates, United States, 2007

State	Rate, %	State	Rate, %	State	Rate, %	State	Rate, %
Alabama	30.3	Illinois	24.9	Montana	21.8	Rhode Island	21.4
Alaska	27.5	Indiana	26.8	Nebraska	26.0	South Carolina	28.4
Arizona	25.4	Iowa	26.9	Nevada	24.1	South Dakota	26.2
Arkansas	28.7	Kansas	26.9	New Hampshire	24.4	Tennessee	30.1
California	22.6	Kentucky	27.4	New Jersey	23.5	Texas	28.1
Colorado	18.7	Louisiana	29.8	New Mexico	24.0	Utah	21.8
Connecticut	21.2	Maine	24.8	New York	25.0	Vermont	21.3
Delaware	27.4	Maryland	25.4	North Carolina	28.0	Virginia	24.3
Washington, DC	21.8	Massachusetts	21.3	North Dakota	26.5	Washington	25.3
Florida	23.6	Michigan	27.7	Ohio	27.5	West Virginia	29.5
Georgia	28.2	Minnesota	25.5	Oklahoma	28.1	Wisconsin	23.7
Hawaii	21.4	Mississippi	32.0	Oregon	25.5	Wyoming	23.7
Idaho	24.5	Missouri	27.5	Pennsylvania	27.1		

Source: Centers for Disease Control and Prevention, Behavioral Risk Factor Surveillance System.

BMI of 30 or higher, continues to increase in children and adults. The prevalence rate of obesity among men in 2006 was 33 percent, and for women it equaled 35.3 percent.[34] The obesity prevalence rate among children and adolescents was 16.3 percent in 2006. It is obvious that obesity is a condition that starts in childhood.[35] To illustrate the alarming trend in increasing prevalence rates, Colorado was the only state in 2007 with an obesity prevalence rate of less than 20 percent. Alabama, Mississippi, and Tennessee had an obesity prevalence rate of 30 percent or higher (Table 12.7).

Obesity increases the risk of developing many serious diseases. These include coronary heart disease, type 2 diabetes, endometrial cancer, breast cancer, colon cancer, hypertension, dyslipidemia, stroke, liver and gallbladder disease, sleep apnea and respiratory tract problems, osteoarthritis, and gynecological problems in women. Health officials are worried about these trends in obesity, and two objectives in the Healthy People 2010 program target obesity. These objectives are to reduce the prevalence rate of overweight and obesity in adults to less than 15 percent and to reduce the prevalence rate of obesity among children and adolescents to less than 5 percent.[36]

Figure 12.1 presents a historical perspective of the trends in overweight and obesity in the United States since 1960. Since 1976, the prevalence of overweight and obesity has dramatically increased in people between the ages of twenty and seventy-four years. The most troubling trend is the increase in

FIGURE 12.1: Overweight and obesity prevalence trend, United States, 1960 to 2004

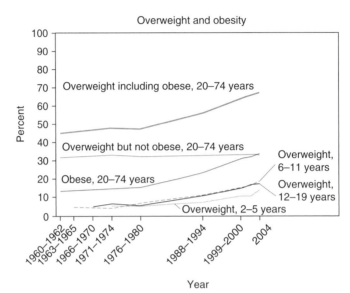

Source: CDC/NCHS, Health, *United States, 2009*, Figure 7. Data from the National Health Examination Survey and the National Health and Nutrition Examination Survey.

the prevalence of overweight in people between the ages of two and nineteen years. This trend indicates the future impact of overweight and obesity in the United States.

Colorectal Cancer

Colorectal cancer is cancer of the colon or rectum. It is the second leading cause of death from cancer in the United States. Deaths from colorectal cancer surpassed 53,000 in 2004, with about 50 percent of deaths in men and women. Colorectal cancer is the most-often diagnosed cancer, with more than 145,000 diagnoses in 2004. It is the third most prevalent cancer diagnosis in both men and women.

Colorectal cancer affects men and women equally in all racial and ethnic groups. Age is a factor, with most cases occurring in people aged fifty years or older. One reason for the number of cases is the lack of screening, which has proved effective in decreasing the serious and fatal effects. In the United States, more than 40 million people older than 50 years do not receive screening for colorectal cancer.[37]

Cervical Cancer

Cervical cancer is a gynecological cancer that begins in the cervix, which is the lower end of the uterus. The cervix connects the uterus to the vagina. Cervical cancer is more prevalent in women thirty years of age and older. In the United States in 2004, almost 12,000 cases of cervical cancer were diagnosed, and about 4,000 women died. All women are at risk for cervical cancer. In 2004, 1,892 women in the United States were told they had cervical cancer, and 3,850 died from the disease.[38]

Cervical cancer is caused by the human papilloma virus, which is transmitted during sexual intercourse. In fact, all women who have sex are at risk for infection from the human papilloma virus. More women are infected than the ones in whom cervical cancer develops. Cervical cancer can be prevented through vaccination and screening. When identified early in its development, cervical cancer survival is high. The screening test, called a Pap smear, is easily performed and accurate and should be done once a year. The Pap smear is used to find precancerous cells, which may change and become cancerous.

Because of screening and vaccinations, the incidence rate of cervical cancer has decreased over the past ten years. There has been a 4 percent decrease in new cases overall. This decrease has been higher in blacks (3.7 percent) and Hispanics (3.6 percent) than in whites (2.5 percent). The greatest decrease has been seen in Asian and Pacific Islanders, who had a 6 percent reduction. This same trend has been seen in cervical cancer deaths, with a 4 percent decrease among all women.[39]

Prostate Cancer

Prostate cancer is the second most prevalent cancer among men (skin cancer being the most common). In the United States in 2004, more than 189,000 men were diagnosed with prostate cancer. Of these, almost 30,000 died. Prostate cancer is the second leading cancer cause of death in men (lung cancer being the leading cancer cause of death), and is the seventh leading cause of death overall.[40] Fortunately, the incidence rate of prostate cancer has not changed since 1995, and prostate cancer deaths have decreased by 4 percent over the past ten years.

The risk factors for prostate cancer are many and diverse. The most important is age: most new cases of prostate cancer are found in men aged sixty-five years and older. Family history is also important. If prostate cancer has occurred in a person's immediate family, his risk of developing the disease increases three times. It is more common in African Americans than in any other racial or ethnic group. In fact, the prostate cancer death rate is highest in African Americans.[41]

Skin Cancer

The most common type of cancer is skin cancer, which mostly occurs as either *basal cell* or *squamous cell carcinoma*. These carcinomas are easily treated and eliminated, but melanoma, another type of skin cancer, is much more severe. In 2004 more than 50,000 new cases were diagnosed in the United States. About 8,000 people died of skin cancer in that year.[42] The incidence rate of melanoma has not changed since 2000 in men and women, but it has increased more than 3 percent in whites since 1981. The death rate for skin cancer has decreased slightly since 1990, with the reduction seen among women. The risk factors for skin cancer differ by the type of carcinoma. These include light skin color, family history, previous skin cancer, exposure to the sun, blue or green eyes, and blond or red hair.[43] Skin cancer can be prevented by protection from the effects of the sun by avoiding exposure, wearing protective clothing, wearing a hat, and using sunglasses and sunscreen.

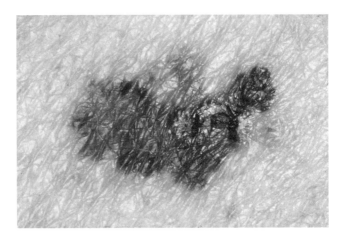

Asthma

Asthma is a lung disease that is most frequently seen in children. The effects of asthma are wheezing, breathlessness, chest tightness, and coughing. About 22 million people in the United States had asthma in 2005, or a 7.7 percent preva-lence rate. The prevalence rate was highest in children (8.9 percent), with a 7.2 percent rate in adults. The highest prevalence rate was in African Americans, American Indians, and Alaska natives, who had a 25 percent rate. The asthma prevalence rate is higher in boys than in girls.

Clinically asthma occurs as episodic attacks. About 12.2 million new people experienced at least one asthma attack in 2005. Of the existing cases of asthma, 55 percent had at least one asthma attack in 2005. As was stated above, the highest asthma attack prevalence rate was seen in children. Women have double the attack rate of men. People living in Puerto Rico had a one-and-a-half times higher attack rate than all other Hispanics.[44]

More than 32 million people have been diagnosed with asthma during their lives. About 23 million of these people were adults. People from Puerto Rico have the highest rate of lifetime asthma among Hispanics. Blacks have the highest rate of lifetime asthma among all races.

Table 12.8 presents the lifetime asthma estimates in the United States. The table shows that there are more than 32 million cases of lifetime asthma. Of these, the majority of cases occurred in adults. The difference between children and adult cases is significant across all races, except for Hispanics. More cases occur in women and whites.[45]

Table 12.9 shows the current cases of asthma in the United States. Currently there are more than 22 million cases of asthma, with more than 16 million adult cases. There are slightly more cases among females than males, with most cases

TABLE 12.8: Lifetime Asthma Population Estimates by Age, United States, 2006

	All Ages	Children (age <18 years)	Adults (18 years and older)
Total	34,132,000	9,876,000	24,256,000
Male	15,953,000	5,875,000	10,078,000
Female	18,179,000	4,001,000	14,178,000
White	23,166,000	5,606,000	17,559,000
Black	4,955,000	1,887,000	3,068,000
Hispanic	4,246,000	1,901,000	2,345,000
Other races	1,755,000	481,000	1,284,000

Source: Centers for Disease Control and Prevention, National Center for Health Statistics, Division of Health Interview Statistics. Data from the National Health Interview Survey, 2006.

TABLE 12.9: Current Asthma Estimates by Age, United States, 2006

	All Ages	Children (age <18 years)	Adults (18 years and older)
Total	22,876,000	6,819,000	16,057,000
Male	10,026,000	4,122,000	5,904,000
Female	12,850,000	2,697,000	10,152,000
White	15,573,000	3,771,000	11,801,000
Black	3,391,000	1,442,000	1,949,000
Hispanic	2,775,000	1,328,000	1,447,000
Other races	1,137,000	278,000	859,000

Source: Centers for Disease Control and Prevention, National Center for Health Statistics, Division of Health Interview Statistics. Data from the National Health Interview Survey, 2006.

TABLE 12.10: Current Asthma Prevalence Rates by Age, Sex, and Race, United States, 2006*

	All Ages	Children (age <18 years)	Adults (18 years and older)
Total	7.8	9.3	7.3
Male	7.0	11.0	5.6
Female	8.6	7.5	8.9
White	7.9	8.8	7.7
Black	9.2	12.7	7.7
Hispanic	6.4	9.0	5.1
Other races	7.1	6.9	7.2

*Percent.
Source: Centers for Disease Control and Prevention, National Center for Health Statistics, Division of Health Interview Statistics. Data from the National Health Interview Survey, 2006.

occurring in whites. Note that almost an equal number of asthma cases occur between Hispanic children and Hispanic adults.

Table 12.10 presents the current asthma prevalence in the United States according to age, sex, and race. The overall prevalence rate is 7.8 percent, with a higher prevalence seen in children. The prevalence rate of females is higher than males overall. But the prevalence rate in male children is much higher than in female children. Blacks have a higher overall prevalence rate, which is even more pronounced in children.[46]

TABLE 12.11: Age-Specific Prevalence Rate of Diagnosed Diabetes per 100 Population by Sex and Race or Ethnicity, 2005*

	0 to 44 Years of Age	45 to 64 Years of Age	65 to 74 Years of Age	75 Years of Age and Older
White male	1.3	10.0	20.0	16.4
White female	1.4	8.6	15.4	13.4
Black male	1.7	16.9	26.6	22.0
Black female	1.7	15.9	28.7	29.1
Hispanic male	1.1	13.3	31.2	22.7
Hispanic female	1.3	15.9	27.7	22.3

*Percent.
Source: Centers for Disease Control and Prevention, National Center for Health Statistics, Division of Health Interview Statistics.

TABLE 12.12: Number of Persons with Diagnosed Diabetes, in Millions, United States, 1990 to 2005

Year	Number	Year	Number
1990	6.6	1998	10.5
1991	6.9	1999	11.1
1992	7.5	2000	12.0
1993	7.6	2001	12.9
1994	8.1	2002	13.6
1995	8.0	2003	14.3
1996	8.8	2004	15.2
1997	9.4	2005	15.8

Source: Centers for Disease Control and Prevention, National Center for Health Statistics, Division of Health Interview Statistics.

Diabetes

Table 12.11 shows the prevalence rate of diagnosed diabetes by age, sex, and race in the United States in 2005. It is clear that diabetes prevalence increases with age, with a slight decrease in the group aged seventy-five years and older. The highest prevalence rate is seen in Hispanic men, closely followed by black women. Whites, both male and female, have the lowest prevalence, with white women having a rate that is almost 50 percent lower than others.

Table 12.12 presents the number of diagnosed cases of diabetes each year, from 1990 to 2005. The number of people diagnosed each year has increased

TABLE 12.13: Crude and Age-Adjusted Prevalence Rates of Diagnosed Diabetes per 100 Population, United States, 1990 to 2005

Year	Crude Rate, %	Age-Adjusted Rate, %	Year	Crude Rate, %	Age-Adjusted Rate, %
1990	2.7	2.9	1998	3.9	4.1
1991	2.8	3.0	1999	4.1	4.2
1992	3.0	3.1	2000	4.4	4.5
1993	3.0	3.2	2001	4.7	4.7
1994	3.1	3.3	2002	4.8	4.9
1995	3.1	3.3	2003	5.0	5.0
1996	3.3	3.5	2004	5.3	5.2
1997	3.5	3.7	2005	5.5	5.3

Source: Centers for Disease Control and Prevention, National Center for Health Statistics, Division of Health Interview Statistics.

steadily, from 6.6 million in 1990 to 15.8 million in 2005. These numbers indicate that diabetes cases have more than doubled since 1990.

In an attempt to better understand the future impact of diabetes, Table 12.13 presents crude and age-adjusted prevalence rates of diagnosed diabetes from 1990 to 2005. After adjusting for changes in the age of the United States population, it is obvious that the prevalence rate of diabetes has continued to increase over the years. In fact, the prevalence rate has almost doubled in the past fifteen years. These numbers and rates indicate that diabetes will be a health problem for many years into the future.

Summary

Epidemiology is involved in our everyday lives more than ever before. Epidemiology plays a major role in terrorism preparedness, especially with the threat of biological agents. Syndromic surveillance is used to monitor bioterrorism.

Chronic diseases represent the leading causes of death today. Heart disease is the number one cause of death, followed by cancers of the lung, breast, prostate, and skin. Obesity is a condition that has become more prevalent across the United States and is linked to diabetes and the risk of death from cancer. Other conditions, such as asthma, are continuing to affect large numbers of people.

Today, in addition to the continuing burden of chronic disease, we are faced with emerging infectious diseases, including H1N1 flu. In fact, several infectious diseases that had become rare over the twentieth century, such as TB, are again raising concerns.

Key Terms

Avian influenza, 234

Basal cell carcinoma, 252

Bird flu, 234

Bovine spongiform encephalopathy (BSE), 238

Disease, 230

Mad cow disease, 238

Methicillin-resistant *Staphylococcus aureus* (MRSA), 236

Squamous cell carcinoma, 252

Syndromic surveillance, 230

Chapter Exercises

1. Using newspaper and Internet sources, research the number of infectious disease outbreaks that have occurred over the past twelve months in your community. Write a short paper describing the outbreaks in terms of duration, cause, and who was affected (include characteristics of the people and the numbers).
2. Name three emerging diseases and list their characteristics.
3. In which state does West Nile virus cause the most concern? Explain your answer.
4. What does the trend in the number of people with diagnosed diabetes indicate for the future? Explain your answer.

Chapter Review

1. The obesity epidemic has begun to disappear over the past ten years. True or False?
2. Obesity increases the risk of
   a. diabetes.
   b. coronary heart disease.
   c. breast cancer.

    d. colon cancer.

    e. all of the above.

    f. none of the above.

3. Asthma is more of a problem in adults than in children. True or False?

4. The most important risk factor for prostate cancer in men is

    a. diet.

    b. lack of exercise.

    c. age.

    d. none of the above.

5. All women are at risk for cervical cancer. True or False?

6. The death rate from heart disease is highest among

    a. Hispanics.

    b. Asians.

    c. whites.

    d. blacks.

7. Breast cancer only affects women. True or False?

8. Lyme disease is transmitted by

    a. mosquitos.

    b. fungi.

    c. ticks.

    d. all of the above.

9. Poliomyelitis can be prevented by vaccination. True or False?

10. A positive skin test for TB indicates

    a. that the person has active tuberculosis.

    b. the person may have been exposed to the tuberculosis bacterium.

    c. more testing is needed.

    d. a and c.

    e. b and c.

Preface

1. *State Public Health Employee Workforce Shortage Report: A Civil Service Recruitment and Retention Crisis*. Arlington, VA: Association of State and Territorial Health Officials; 2004.
2. Honoré PA, Graham G, Garcia J, and Morris W. A call to action: Public health and community college partnerships to educate the workforce and promote health equity. *Journal of Public Health Management and Practice*. 2008; 14(56) Suppl:S82–S84.

Chapter One

1. Mausner JS and Kramer S. *Epidemiology: An Introductory Text*. 2nd ed. Philadelphia, Wiley; 1985.
2. Last JM, ed. *A Dictionary of Epidemiology*. 4th ed. New York: Oxford University Press; 2000.
3. Centers for Disease Control and Prevention. Smallpox eradication. Available at: http://www.cdc.gov/Features/SmallpoxEradication. Accessed Sept. 23, 2009.
4. National Institute of Neurological Disorders and Stroke. Reye's syndrome. Available at: http://www.ninds.nih.gov/disorders/reyes_syndrome/reyes_syndrome.htm. Accessed Sept. 23, 2009.
5. Centers for Disease Control and Prevention. Legionella. Available at: http://www.cdc.gov/legionella/index.htm. Accessed Sept. 23, 2009.
6. Institute of Medicine, Committee for the Study of the Future of Public Health, Division of Health Care Services. *The Future of Public Health*. Washington, DC: National Academy Press; 1988.
7. *Directions for Health: New Approaches to Population Health Research and Practice*. The Leeds Declaration. Leeds, England: Nuffield Institute for Health, University of Leeds; 1993.
8. Susser M. Epidemiology today: "A thought-tormented world." *International Journal of Epidemiology*. 1989; 18:481–488.

9. Lilienfeld D and Lilienfeld A. Epidemiology: A retrospective study. *American Journal of Epidemiology*. 1977; 106:445–449.

10. Kindig DA. *Purchasing Population Health*. Ann Arbor: University of Michigan Press; 1997.

Chapter Two

1. Singer C and Underwood EA. *A Short History of Medicine*. 2nd ed. Oxford, England: Clarendon Press; 1962.

2. Newcomb RD and Marshall ED. *Public Health and Community Optometry*. 2nd ed. Boston: Butterworth; 1990.

3. Brier B. Infectious diseases in ancient Egypt. *Infectious Disease Clinics of North America*. 2004; 18(1):17–27.

4. Robinson OF. *Ancient Rome: City Planning and Administration*. London: Routledge; 1991.

5. Ackerknecht EH. *A Short History of Medicine*. Baltimore: Johns Hopkins University Press; 1982.

6. Dupaquier J and Dupaquier M. *Historie de la Demographie [History of Demography]*. Paris: Perrin; 1985.

7. Meynell GG. *Materials for a Biography of Thomas Sydenham (1624–1689): A New Survey of Public and Private Archives*. Folkestone, England: Winterdown Books; 1988.

8. Eyler JM. The conceptual origins of William Farris epidemiology: Numerical methods and social thought in the 1930s. In: Lilienfeld AM, ed. *Time, Persons and Places*. Baltimore: Johns Hopkins University Press; 1980.

9. Lilienfeld DE. John Snow: The first hired gun? *American Journal of Epidemiology*. 2000; 125(1):4–9.

10. Collins CH. John Snow: On the mode of communication of cholera. *Medical Sciences History*. 2003; 19:12–13.

11. Winkelstein W Jr. A new perspective of John Snow's communicable disease theory. *American Journal of Epidemiology*. 1995; 142:53–59.

12. *Smoking and Health: Report of the Advisory Committee to the Surgeon General of the Public Health Service*. Washington, DC: United States Public Health Service, publication No. 1103, 1964.

13. Leventhal T and Brooks-Gunn J. Moving to opportunity: An experimental study of neighborhood effects on mental health. *American Journal of Public Health*. 2003; 93:1576–1582.

14. Gordon T, Castelli WP, Hjortland MC, Kannel WB, and Dawber TR. Diabetes, blood lipids, and the role of obesity in coronary heart disease risk for women: The Framingham study. *Annals of Internal Medicine*. 1977; 87:393–397.

15. Kannel WB and Benjamin EJ. Current perceptions of the epidemiology of atrial fibrillation. *Cardiology Clinics*. 2009; 27(1):13–24, vii.

16. Voors AW, Foster TA, Frerichs RR, Webber LS, Berenson GS. Studies of blood pressures in children, ages 5–14 years, in a total biracial community: The Bogalusa Heart Study. *Circulation*. 1976; 54:319–327.

17. Nguyen QM, Srinivasan SR, Xu JH, Chen W, and Berenson GS. Changes in risk variables of metabolic syndrome since childhood in pre-diabetic and type 2 diabetic subjects: The Bogalusa Heart Study. *Diabetes Care.* 2008; 31(10):2044–2049.

Chapter Three

1. World Health Organization. Preamble to Constitution of the World Organization, *Official Records of the World Health Organization.* 1948; (2):100.
2. Pope John Paul II Conference of the International Federations of Catholic Health Care Workers, Feb. 2000; Vatican City.
3. Lalonde M. *A New Perspective on the Health of Canadians.* Ottawa, Toronto: Minister of Supply and Services; 1974.
4. McHorney CA. Health status assessment methods for adults: Past accomplishments and future challenges. *Annual Review of Public Health.* 1999; 20:309–335.
5. Stokols D. Establishing and maintaining healthy environments: Toward a social ecology of health promotion. *American Psychologist.* 1992; 47:6–22.
6. Idler EL and Benyamini Y. Self-reported health and mortality: A review of twenty-seven community studies. *Journal of Health and Social Behavior.* 1997; 38:21–37.
7. Centers for Disease Control and Prevention. *Measuring Healthy Days.* Atlanta: Centers for Disease Control and Prevention; 2000.
8. Fletcher RH, Fletcher SW, and Wagner EH. *Clinical Epidemiology: The Essentials.* 2nd ed. Baltimore: Williams & Wilkins; 1988.
9. Harris MI, Flegal KM, Cowie CC, Eberhardt MS, Goldstein DE, Little RR, Weidmeyer HM, and Byrd-Holt DD. Prevalence of diabetes, impaired fasting glucose, and impaired glucose tolerance in U.S. adults. *Diabetes Care.* 1998; 21:518–524.
10. Eriksson KF and Lindgarde F. Prevention of type 2 (non-insulin-dependent) diabetes mellitus by diet and physical exercise: The 6-year Malmo Feasibility Study. *Diabetologia.* 1991; 34:891–898.
11. American Diabetes Association. Consensus statement: The pharmacologic treatment of hyperglycemia in NIDDM. *Diabetes Care.* 1996; 19:S354–S361.
12. Descotes J. *Immunotoxicology of Drugs and Chemicals.* Amsterdam: Elsevier; 1988.
13. Duesberg PH and Rasnick D. The AIDS dilemma: Drug diseases blamed on a passenger virus. *Genetica.* 1998; 104:85–132.
14. Jain VK and Chandra RK. Does nutritional deficiency predispose to acquired immunodeficiency syndrome? *Nutrition Research.* 1984; 4:537–542.
15. Lauritsen J. *Poison by Prescription: The AZT Story.* New York: Asklepios; 1990.
16. Chandra RK. Nutrition, immunity and infection: Present knowledge and future directions. *Lancet.* 1983; 1(8326Pt 1):688–691.
17. Root-Bernstein RS and Hobbs de Witt S. Semen alloantigen and lymphocytotoxic antibodies in AIDS and ICL. *Genetica.* 1995; 95:133–156.
18. World Bank. *Confronting AIDS: Public Priorities in a Global Epidemic.* A World Bank Policy Research Report; 1999.

19. Fischbein A and Tarcher AB. Disorders of the immune system. In: Tarcher AB, ed. *Principles and Practice of Environmental Medicine*. New York: Plenum Medical Book Co.; 1992.

20. Shuper PA, Neuman M, Kanteres F, Balliunas D, Joharchi N, and Rehm J. Causal considerations on alcohol and HIV/AIDS: A systematic review. *Alcohol and Alcoholism*. 2010; 45(2):159–166.

21. Giraldo RA. AIDS and stressors II: A proposal for the pathogenesis of AIDS stressors. In: *AIDS and Stressors*. Medellín, Colombia: Impresos Begón; 1997.

22. Papadopulos-Eleopulos E. Reappraisal of AIDS—is the oxidation induced by the risk factors the primary cause? *Medical Hypothesis*. 1988; 25:151–162.

23. Friis R and Sellers T. *Epidemiology for Public Health Practice*. 4th Ed. Sudbury, MA: Jones and Bartlett; 2009.

24. *Hippocrates*. vol. V. Potter, P., trans. Cambridge, MA: Harvard University Press, 1988.

25. Bradford-Hill A. The environment and disease: Association or causation? *Proceedings of the Royal Society of Medicine*. 1965; 58:295–300.

26. Rothman KJ. *Modern Epidemiology*. Boston: Little Brown; 1986.

27. Mausner JS and Kramer S. *Epidemiology: An Introductory Text*. 2nd ed. Philadelphia: Saunders; 1985.

Chapter Four

1. Daniel W. *Biostatistics: A Foundation for Analysis in Health Sciences*. 6th ed. New York: Wiley; 1995.

2. Li L, Young D, Xiao S, Zhou X, and Zhou L. Psychometric properties of the WHO Quality of Life questionnaire (WHOQOL-100) in patients with chronic diseases and their caregivers in China. *Bulletin of the World Health Organization*. 2004; 82(7):493–502.

3. Hancox JG, Sheridan SC, Feldman SR, and Fleischer AB. Seasonal variation of dermatologic disease in the USA: A study of office visits from 1990 to 1998. *International Journal of Dermatology*. 2004; 43:6–11.

4. Centers for Disease Control and Prevention; Lyytikäinen O, Turunen H, Sund R, Rasinperä M, Könönen E, Ruutu P, et al. Hospitalizations and deaths related to *Clostridium difficile* infection, Finland, 1996–2004. *Emerging Infectious Diseases* [online serial]. Available at: http://www.cdc.gov/EID/content/15/5/761.htm. Accessed May 2009.

5. Ford ES, Mannino DM, Redd SC, Moriarty DG, and Mokdad AH. Determinants of quality of life among people with asthma: Findings from the Behavioral Risk Factor Surveillance System. *Journal of Asthma*. 2004; 41:327–336.

6. Grunbaum JA, Kann L, Kinchen S, Ross J, Hawkins J, Lowry R, Harris WA, McManus T, Chyen D, and Collins J. Youth risk behavior surveillance: United States, 2003. *MMWR Surveillance Summaries*. 2004; 53:1–96.

7. Gregg EW, Cheng YJ, Cadwell BS, Imperatore G, Williams DE, Flegal KM, Venkat Narayan KM, and Williamson DF. Secular changes in cardiovascular disease risk

factors according to body mass index in US adults. *Journal of the American Medical Association*. 2005; 293:1868–1874.

Chapter Five

1. U.S. Cancer Statistics Working Group. *United States Cancer Statistics: 1999–2004 Incidence and Mortality Web-Based Report*. Atlanta: U.S. Department of Health and Human Services, Centers for Disease Control and Prevention and National Cancer Institute; 2007.
2. Centers for Disease Control and Prevention. Behavioral Risk Factor Surveillance System, 2007. Available at: http://www.cdc.gov/brfss. Accessed: Jan. 12, 2010.
3. National Health and Nutrition Examination Surveys, National Center for Health Statistics, Centers for Disease Control and Prevention, 2004.
4. Freeman J and Hutchison GB. Prevalence, incidence, and duration. *American Journal of Epidemiology*. 1980; 112:707–723.
5. National Immunization Program, Centers for Disease Control and Prevention. *Epidemiology and Prevention of Vaccine-Preventable Diseases*. 11th ed. Atlanta: Centers for Disease Control and Prevention; 2009.
6. National Center for Chronic Disease Prevention and Health Promotion, Centers for Disease Control and Prevention. *Measuring Healthy Days: Population Assessment of Health-Related Quality of Life*. Atlanta: Centers for Disease Control and Prevention; 2000.
7. Gardner JW and Sanborn JS. Years of potential life lost: What does it measure? *Epidemiology*. 1990; 1(4):322–329.
8. Fos PJ and Fine DJ. *Designing Health Care for Populations*. San Francisco: Jossey-Bass; 2000.

Chapter Six

1. Sirard JR, Ainsworth BE, McIver KL, and Pate RR. Prevalence of active commuting at urban and suburban elementary schools in Columbia, SC. *American Journal of Public Health*. 2005; 95:236–237.
2. Chang S, Crothers C, and Lamm S. Pediatric neurobehavioral decreases in Nevada counties with respect to perchlorate in drinking water: An ecological inquiry. *Birth Defects Research Plan A: Clinical and Molecular Toxicology*. 2003; 67:886–892.
3. Kerani RP, Handcock MS, and Handsfield KK. Comparative geographic concentrations of 4 sexually transmitted diseases. *American Journal of Public Health*. 2005; 95:324–330.
4. *The Amsterdam Cohort Studies on HIV Infection Annual Report, 2006*. Amsterdam: Amsterdam Health Service; 2007.

5. Meyers Jensen KC and Menitove JE. A historical cohort study of the effect of lowering body iron through blood donation on incident cardiac events. *Transfusion*. 2002; 42(9):1135–1139.

6. Jiang HJ, Andrews R, Stryer D, and Friedman B. Racial/ethnic disparities in potentially preventable readmissions: The case of diabetes. *American Journal of Public Health*. 2005; 95:1561–1567.

7. Dell JL, Whitman S, Shan AM, Silva A, and Ansell D. Smoking in 6 diverse Chicago communities: A population study. *American Journal of Public Health*. 2005; 95:1036–1042.

8. Anazalone DA, Anzalone FL, and Fos PJ. High density lipoprotein-cholesterol: Determining hygienic factors for intervention. *Journal of Occupational and Environmental Medicine*. 1995; 37(7):856–861.

9. Wechsler H and Nelson TF. What we have learned from the Harvard School of Public Health Alcohol College Study: focusing attention on college student alcohol consumption and the environmental conditions that promote it. *Journal of Studies on Alcohol and Drugs*. 2008; 69(4):481–490.

10. Wechsler H, Lee JE, Nelson TF, and Lee H. Drinking and driving among college students: The influence of alcohol-control policies. *American Journal of Preventive Medicine*. 2003; 25(3):212–213.

11. Roach M 3rd, Lu J, Pilepich MV, Asbell SO, Mohiuddin M, and Grignon D. Race and survival of men treated for prostate cancer on Radiation Therapy Oncology Group phase III randomized trials. *Journal of Urology*. 2003; 169(1):245–250.

12. Loibl S, von Minckwitz G, Harbeck N, Janni W, Elling D, Kaufmann M, Eggemann H, Nekljudova V, Sommer H, Kiechle M, and Kümmel S. Clinical feasibility of (neo)adjuvant taxane-based chemotherapy in older patients: Analysis of >4,500 patients from four German randomized breast cancer trials. *Breast Cancer Research*. 2008; 10(5):R77.

13. Hurria A, Hurria A, Brogan K, Panageas KS, Pearce C, Norton L, Jakubowski A, Howard J, and Hudis C. Effect of creatinine clearance on patterns of toxicity in older patients receiving adjuvant chemotherapy for breast cancer. *Drugs and Aging*. 2005; 22(9):785–791.

14. Reynolds JK and Levien TL. Quality-of-life assessment in phase III clinical trials of gemcitabine in non-small-cell lung cancer. *Drugs and Aging*. 2008; 25(11):893–911.

Chapter Seven

1. Magann EF, Chauhan SP, Mobley JA, Klausen JH, Martin JN Jr, and Morrison JC. Risk factors for secondary arrest of labor among women >41 weeks' gestation with an unfavorable cervix undergoing membrane sweeping for cervical ripening. *International Journal of Gynaecological Obstetrics*. 1999; 65(1):1–5.

2. Egberts ACG, Meyboom RHB, and van Puijenbroek EP. Use of measures of disproportionality in pharmacovigilance. *Drug Safety*. 2002; 26:453–458.

3. Hauben M and Zhou X. Quantitative methods in pharmacovigilance. *Drug Safety*. 2003; 26:159–186.

Chapter Eight

1. McFarland JM, Baddour LM, Nelson JE, Elkins SK, Craven RB, Cropp BC, Chang GJ, Grindstaff AD, Craig ASM, and Smith RJ. Imported yellow fever in a United States citizen. *Clinical Infectious Diseases.* 1997; 25(5):1143–1147.

2. Centers for Disease Control and Prevention. 1993 revised classification system for HIV77 infection and expanded surveillance case definition for AIDS among adolescents and adults. *Morbidity and Mortality Weekly Report.* 1992; 41(No. RR-17).

3. Centers for Disease Control and Prevention. Legionnaires' disease outbreak associated with a grocery store mist machine—Louisiana, 1989. *Morbidity and Mortality Weekly Report.* 1990; 39:108–110.

4. Mostashari F, Bunning ML, Kitsutani PT, Singer DA, Nash D, Cooper MJ, Katz N, Liljebjelke KA, Biggerstaff BJ, Fine AD, Layton MC, Mullin SM, Johnson AJ, Martin DA, Hayes EB, and Campbell GL. Epidemic West Nile encephalitis, New York, 1999: Results of a household-based seroepidemiological survey. *Lancet.* 2001; 358(9278):261–264.

Chapter Nine

1. Rose G. *The Strategy of Preventive Medicine.* Oxford, England: Oxford University Press; 1992.

2. Berkman LF and Kawachi I, eds. *Social Epidemiology.* New York: Oxford University Press; 2000.

3. Zheng Y, Ye DQ, Pan HF, Li WX, Li LH, Li J, Li XP, and Xu JH. Influence of social support on health-related quality of life in patients with systemic lupus erythematosus. *Clinical Rheumatology.* 2009; 28(3):265–269 [published online Nov. 11, 2008].

4. Wellman B and Berkowitz SD, eds. *Social Structures: A Network Approach.* Cambridge, England: Cambridge University Press; 1988.

5. Smith KP and Christakis NA. Social networks and health. *Annual Review of Sociology.* 2008; 34:405–429.

6. Clegg LX, Reichman ME, Miller BA, Hankey BF, Singh GK, Lin YD, Goodman MT, Lynch CF, Schwartz SM, Chen VW, Bernstein L, Gomez SL, Graff JJ, Lin CC, Johnson NJ, and Edwards BK. Impact of socioeconomic status on cancer incidence and stage at diagnosis: Selected findings from the surveillance, epidemiology, and end results: National Longitudinal Mortality Study. *Cancer Causes and Control.* 2009 May; 20(4):417–435 [published online Nov. 12, 2008].

7. Marmot MG, Shipley MJ, Hemingway H, Head J, and Brunner EJ. Biological and behavioural explanations of social inequalities in coronary heart disease: The Whitehall II study. *Diabetologia.* 2008; 51(11):1980–1988 [published online Sept. 6, 2008].

8. Centers for Disease Control and Prevention. Cigarette smoking among adults: United States, 1994. *Morbidity and Mortality Weekly Report.* 1996; 45:588–590.

9. Marmot M. The influence of income on health: Views of an epidemiologist. Does money really matter? Or is it a marker for something else? *Health Affairs (Millwood)*. 2002; 21:31–46.

10. Subramanian SV and Kawachi I. Wage poverty, earned income inequality, and health. In: Heymann J, ed. *Global Inequalities at Work*. New York: Oxford University Press; 2003:165–187.

11. Wagstaff A and van Doorslaer E. Income inequality and health: What does the literature tell us? *Annual Review of Public Health*. 2000; 21:543–567.

12. Rodgers GB. Income and inequality as determinants of mortality: an international cross-section analysis. *Population Studies (Cambridge)*. 1979; 33:343–351.

13. Blakely TA, Kennedy BP, Glass R, and Kawachi I. What is the lag time between income inequality and health status? *Journal of Epidemiology and Community Health*. 2000; 54:318–319.

14. Diez-Roux AV, Link BG, and Northridge ME. A multilevel analysis of income inequality and cardiovascular disease risk factors. *Social Science and Medicine*. 2000; 50(5):673–687.

15. Kennedy BP, Kawashi I, and Prothrow-Stith D. Income distribution and mortality: Cross-sectional ecologic study of the Robin Hood Index in the United States. *British Medical Journal*. 1996; 312:1004–1007.

16. Skodova Z, Nagyova I, van Dijk JP, Sudzinova A, Vargova H, Studencan M, and Reijneveld SA. Socioeconomic differences in psychosocial factors contributing to coronary heart disease: A review. *Journal of Clinical Psychology in Medical Settings*. 2008; 15(3):204–213.

17. Zeka A, Melly SJ, and Schwartz J. The effects of socioeconomic status and indices of physical environment on reduced birth weight and preterm births in Eastern Massachusetts. *Environmental Health*. 2008; 7:60.

18. Stingone JA and Claudio L. Disparities in allergy testing and health outcomes among urban children with asthma. *Journal of Allergy and Clinical Immunology*. 2008; 122(4):748–753.

19. Lopez-McKee G, McNeill JA, Bader J, and Morales P. Comparison of factors affecting repeat mammography screening of low-income Mexican American women. *Oncology Nursing Forum*. 2008; 35(6):941–947.

20. Ben-Shlomo Y and Kuh D. A life course approach to chronic disease epidemiology: Conceptual models, empirical challenges and interdisciplinary perspectives. *International Journal of Epidemiology*. 2002; 31:285–293.

21. Heslop P, Smith GD, Macleod J, and Hart C. The socioeconomic position of employed women, risk factors and mortality. *Social Science and Medicine*. 2001; 53:477–485.

22. Galobardes B, Lynch JW, and Smith GD. Childhood socioeconomic circumstances and cause-specific mortality in adulthood: Systematic review and interpretation. *Epidemiologic Reviews*. 2004; 26:7–21.

23. Berenson GS, Srinivasan SR, Freedman DS, Radhakrishnamurthy B, and Dalferes ER Jr. Atherosclerosis and its evolution in children. *American Journal of the Medical Sciences*. 1987; 294(6):429–440.

24. Holman RL, McGill HCJ, Strong JP, and Geer JC. The natural history of athero-sclerosis: The early aortic lesions as seen in New Orleans in the middle of the 20th century. *American Journal of Pathology.* 1958; 34:209–235.

25. Burke JP, Williams K, Gaskill SP, Hazuda HP, Haffner SM, and Stern MP. Rapid rise in the incidence of type 2 diabetes from 1987 to 1996: Results from the San Antonio Heart Study. *Archives of Internal Medicine.* 1999; 159:1450–1456.

26. Cowie CC and Eberhardt MS. Sociodemographic characteristics of persons with diabetes. In: Harris MI, Cowie CC, Stern MP, et al., eds. *Diabetes in America.* 2nd ed. Bethesda, MD: National Institutes of Health, 1995:85–116.

27. Brown AF, Gross AG, Gutierrez PR, Jiang L, Shapiro MF, and Mangione CM. Income-related differences in the use of evidence-based therapies in older persons with diabetes mellitus in for-profit managed care. *Journal of the American Geriatrics Society.* 2003; 51:665–670.

28. Connolly V and Kesson CM. Socio-economic status and membership of the British Diabetic Association in Scotland. *Diabetic Medicine.* 1996; 13:898–901.

29. Shi L and Starfield B. Primary care, income inequality, and self-rated health in the United States: a mixed-level analysis. *International Journal of Health Services.* 2000; 30:541–555.

30. Baker RS, Watkins NL, Wilson MR, Bazargan M, and Flowers CW Jr. Demographic and clinical characteristics of patients with diabetes presenting to an urban public hospital ophthalmology clinic. *Ophthalmology.* 1998; 105:1373–1379.

31. Beckles GL, Engelgau MM, Narayan KM, Herman WH, Aubert RE, and Williamson DF. Population-based assessment of the level of care among adults with diabetes in the U.S. *Diabetes Care.* 1998; 21:1432–1438.

32. Koopman JS, Longini IM Jr. The ecological effects of individual exposures and nonlinear disease dynamics in populations. *American Journal of Public Health.* 1994; 84:836–842.

33. Berkman LF and Glass T. Social integration, social networks, social support, and health. In: Berkman LF and Kawachi I, eds. *Social Epidemiology.* New York: Oxford University Press; 2000:137–173.

34. Friedman SR, Kottiri BJ, Neaigus A, Curtis R, Vermund SH, and Des Jarlais DC. Network-related mechanisms may help explain long-term HIV-1 seroprevalence levels that remain high but do not approach population-group saturation. *American Journal of Epidemiology.* 2000; 152:913–922.

35. Laumann EO and Youm Y. Racial/ethnic group differences in the prevalence of sexually transmitted diseases in the United States: A network explanation. *Sexually Transmitted Diseases.* 1999; 26:250–261.

36. Poundstone KE, Strathdee SA, and Celentano DD. The social epidemiology of human immunodeficiency virus/acquired immunodeficiency syndrome. *Epidemiologic Reviews.* 2004; 26:22–35.

37. Lorant V, Deliège D, Eaton W, Robert A, Philippot P, and Ansseau M. Socioeconomic inequalities in depression: a meta-analysis. *American Journal of Epidemiology.* 2003; 157:98–112.

38. Eaton W, Dryman A, and Weissman MM. Panic and phobia. In: Robins LN and Regier DA, eds. *Psychiatric Disorders in America: The Epidemiologic Catchment Area Study*. New York: Free Press; 1991:155–179.

39. Nestadt G, Bienvenu OJ, Cai G, Samuels J, and Eaton WW. Incidence of obsessive-compulsive disorder in adults. *Journal of Nervous and Mental Disease*. 1998; 186:401–406.

40. Galea S, Nandi A, and Vlahov D. The social epidemiology of substance use. *Epidemiologic Reviews*. 2004; 26:36–52.

41. Conwell LS, O'Callaghan MJ, Andersen MJ, Bor W, Najman JM, and Williams GM. Early adolescent smoking and a web of personal and social disadvantage. *Journal of Paediatrics and Child Health*. 2003; 39:580–585.

42. Dawson DA. The link between family history and early onset alcoholism: Earlier initiation of drinking or more rapid development of dependence? *Journal of Studies on Alcohol*. 2000; 61:637–646.

43. Olds RS and Thombs DL. The relationship of adolescent perceptions of peer norms and parent involvement to cigarette and alcohol use. *Journal of School Health*. 2001; 71:223–228.

44. Levy SJ and Pierce JP. Predictors of marijuana use and uptake among teenagers in Sydney, Australia. *International Journal of Addiction*. 1990; 25:1179–1193.

45. von Sydow K, Lieb R, Pfister H, Höfler M, and Wittchen HU. What predicts incident use of cannabis and progression to abuse and dependence? A 4-year prospective examination of risk factors in a community sample of adolescents and young adults. *Drug and Alcohol Dependence*. 2002; 1:49–64.

46. Miller DS and Miller TQ. A test of socioeconomic status as a predictor of initial marijuana use. *Addictive Behaviors*. 1997; 22:479–489.

47. Sriniasan S, O'Fallon LR, and Dearry A. Creating healthy communities, healthy homes, healthy people: Initiating a research agenda on the built environment and public health. *American Journal of Public Health*. 2003; 93(9):1446–1450.

48. Frumkin H. Healthy places: exploring the evidence. *American Journal of Public Health*. 2003; 93(9):1451–1456.

49. Leventhal T and Brooks-Gunn J. Moving to opportunity: An experimental study of neighborhood effects on mental health. *American Journal of Public Health*. 2003; 93(9):1576–1582.

50. Grafova IB, Freedman VA, Kumar R, and Rogowski J. Neighborhoods and obesity in later life. *American Journal of Public Health*. 2008; 98(11):2065–2071.

51. Bell JF, Wilson JS, and Liu GC. Neighborhood greenness and 2-year changes in body mass index in children and youth. *American Journal of Preventive Medicine*. 2008; 35(6):547–553.

52. Centers for Disease Control and Prevention. *Physical Activity and Health: A Report of the Surgeon General*. National Center for Chronic Disease Prevention and Health Promotion, 1996. Available at: http://www.cdc.gov/nccdphp/sgr/index.htm. Accessed: Jan. 12, 2010.

53. Sallis JF, Bauman A, and Pratt M. Environmental and policy interventions to promote physical activity. *American Journal of Preventive Medicine*. 1998; 15:379–397.

54. Giles-Corti B and Donovan R. Relative influences of individual, social environmental, and physical environmental correlates of walking. *American Journal of Public Health*. 2003; 93(9):1583–1589.

55. World Health Organization. *Transport, Environment, and Health*. 1999. Available at: http://siteresources.worldbank.org/INTTSR/Resources/Transport_health &environment.pdf. Accessed: Jan. 12, 2010.

56. McCarthy M. Transport and health. In: *Social Determinants of Health*. Oxford, England: Oxford University Press; 1999:132–154.

57. Pucher J and Leferve C. *The Urban Transport Crisis in Europe and North America*. London: Macmillan; 1996.

58. Pucher J. Transportation paradise: Realm of the nearly perfect automobile? *Transportation Quarterly*. 1999; 53(3):115–120.

Chapter Ten

1. Mokdad AH, Marks JS, Stroup DF, and Gerberding JL. Actual causes of death in the United States, 2000. *Journal of the American Medical Association*. 2004; 291:1238–1245.

2. Goldston SE, ed. *Concepts of Primary Prevention: A Framework for Program Development*. Sacramento: California Department of Mental Health; 1987.

3. Spasoff JM, Harris SS, and Thuriaux MC, eds. *A Dictionary of Epidemiology*. 4th ed. New York: Oxford University Press; 2001.

4. Hebel JR and McCarter RJ. *Study Guide to Epidemiology and Biostatistics*. 6th ed. Sudbury, MA: Jones & Bartlett; 2006.

5. Friis RH and Sellers TA. *Epidemiology for Public Health Practice*. 2nd ed. Gaithersburg, MD: Aspen; 1999.

6. Andriole GL, Levin DL, Crawford ED, Gelmann EP, Pinsky PF, Chia D, Kramer BS, Reding D, Church TR, Grubb RL, Izmirlian G, Ragard LR, Clapp JD, Prorok PC, and Gohagan JK. Prostate cancer screening in the Prostate, Lung, Colorectal and Ovarian (PLCO) Cancer Screening Trial: Findings from the initial screening round of a randomized trial. *Journal of the National Cancer Institute*. 2005 Mar 16; 97:433–438.

7. Mausner JS and Kramer S. *Epidemiology: An Introductory Text*. 2nd ed. Philadelphia: Saunders; 1985.

Chapter Eleven

1. Marmot MG, Bobak M, and Smith GD. Explanations for social inequalities in health. In: Amick BC, Levine S, Tarlov AR, and Walsh DC, eds. *Society and Health*. New York: Oxford University Press; 1995.

2. MacQueen KM, McLellan E, Metzger DS, Kegeles S, Strauss RP, Scotti R, Blanchard L, and Trotter RT. What is community? An evidence-based definition

for participatory public health. *American Journal of Public Health*. 2001; 91(12): 1929–1938.

3. Witmer A. Community health workers: Integral members of the health care work force. *American Journal of Public Health*. 1995; 85:1055–1058.

4. Snedley BD, Stith AY, and Nelson AR, eds. *Unequal Treatment: Confronting Racial and Ethnic Disparities in Health Care*. Washington, DC: Institute of Medicine; 2002.

5. Walters KL and Simoni JM. Reconceptualizing native women's health: An "indigenous" stress-coping model. *American Journal of Public Health*. 2002; 92:520–524.

6. DiClemente RJ, Crosby RA, and Kegler MC. *Emerging Theories in Health Promotion Practice and Research*. San Francisco: Jossey-Bass; 2002.

7. Wiggins N and Borbon A. Core roles and competencies of community health advisors. chap. 3. *The National Community Health Advisor Study: Weaving the Future*. Tucson: University of Arizona Press; 1998.

8. Conner K. New and emerging roles for community health workers. Abstract presentation, American Public Health Association annual meeting, San Diego, 2008.

9. Martinez ACH, Somoza C, and Sabo S. Mariposa Casas Program: Promotora led home based asthma management for U.S. Mexico border families living with asthma. Abstract presentation, American Public Health Association annual meeting, San Diego, 2008.

10. Moore AM, Newton N, Mora S, and Hasbun G. Moving toward Barrios Saludables: Lessons learned from promotora interventions in Latino neighborhoods. Abstract presentation, American Public Health Association annual meeting, San Diego, 2008.

11. Murray CJL and Evans DB. *Health Systems Performance Assessment: Debates, Methods and Empiricism*. Geneva: World Health Organization; 2003.

12. Alter C and Egan M. Logic modeling: A tool for teaching critical thinking in social work practice. *Journal of Social Work Education*. 1997; 33(1):85–102.

13. Coffman J. Learning from logic models: An example of a family/school partnership. Harvard Family Research Project, 1999. Available at: http://www.hfrp.org/ publications-resources/publications-series/Accessed: Jan. 15, 2010.

14. Alter C and Murty S. Logic modeling: A tool for teaching practice evaluation. *Journal of Social Work Education*. 1997; 33(1):103–118.

15. McLaughlin JA and Jordan GB. Logic models: A tool for telling your program's performance story. *Evaluation and Planning*. 1999; 22:65–72.

16. Millar A, Simeone RS, and Carnevale JT. Logic models: A systems tool for performance management. *Evaluation and Program Planning*. 2001; 24:73–81.

17. Veney JE and Kaluzny AD. *Evaluation and Decision Making for Health Services*. 2nd ed. Ann Arbor, MI: Health Administration Press; 1991.

18. Scriven M. The methodology of evaluation. In: Tyler RW, Gagne RM, and Scriven M, eds. *Perspective of Curriculum Evaluation*. Chicago: Rand McNally; 1967.

19. Hulton LJ. An evaluation of a school-based teenage pregnancy prevention program using a logic model framework. *Journal of School Nursing*. 2007; 23(2): 104–110.

20. Kretz LS, Nicholson J, Tait EO, Hubbard A, Friar WW, and Balkovich J. Participation at an urban community senior center: Results of an outreach program designed to maximize use by low income seniors. Abstract presentation, American Public Health Association annual meeting, San Diego, 2008.

21. Riley-Jacome MF and Gallant M. Development and implementation of a community based walking club leader training: Increasing social support for physical activity. Abstract presentation, American Public Health Association annual meeting, San Diego, 2008.

22. Pei X, Goetzel RZ, Short ME, Roemer EC, Luisi D, Quitoni K, Tabrizi MJ, Liss-Levinson RC, and Samoly DK. Two year evaluation of a public-private partnership for a health promotion program at the workplace. Abstract presentation, American Public Health Association annual meeting, San Diego, 2008.

23. Ellickson PL, McCafferty DF, Ghosh-Dastidar B, and Longshore DL. New inroads in preventing adolescent drug use: Results from a large-scale trial of Project ALERT in middle schools. *American Journal of Public Health.* 2003; 93(11):1830–1836.

24. *Healthy People 2010.* vol. II: *Objectives for Improving Health*, part B. Rockville, MD: U.S. Department of Health and Human Services, Centers for Disease Control and Prevention, Health Resources and Services Administration, Indian Health Service, National Institutes of Health; 2000.

25. Gamm LD, Hutchinson LL, Dabney BJ, and Dorsey AM, eds. *Rural Healthy People 2010: A Companion Document to Healthy People 2010.* vol. 1. College Station: Texas A&M University System Health Science Center, School of Rural Public Health, Southwest Rural Health Research Center; 2003.

26. Baker EL and Koplan J. Strengthening the nation's public health infrastructure: Historic challenge, unprecedented opportunity. *Health Affairs (Millwood).* 2002; 21(6):15–27.

27. Grad FP. *The Public Health Law Manual.* 3rd ed. Washington, DC: American Public Health Association; 2004.

28. Lister S. *An Overview of the U.S. Public Health System in the Context of Emergency Preparedness.* Washington, DC: Congressional Research Service, Library of Congress; 2005.

29. Beitsch LM, Brooks RG, Grigg M, and Menachemi N. Structure and functions of state public health agencies. *American Journal of Public Health.* 2006; 96(1):167–172.

Chapter Twelve

1. Bravata DM, McDonald KM, Smith WM, Rydzak C, Szeto H, Buckeridge DL, Haberland C, and Owens DK. Systematic review: Surveillance systems for early detection of bioterrorism-related diseases. *Annals of Internal Medicine.* 2004; 140(11):910–922.

2. Wagner MM, Tsui F, Espino JU, Dato VM, Sittig DF, Caruana RA, McGinnis LF, Deerfield DW, Druzdzel MJ, and Fridsma DB. The emerging science of very early detection of disease outbreaks. *Journal of Public Health Management Practice.* 2001; 7:51–59.

3. Buehler JW, Berkelman RL, Hartley DM, and Peters CJ. Syndromic surveillance and bioterrorism-related epidemics. *Emerging Infectious Diseases.* 2003; 9(10): 1197–1204.

4. Fos PJ, McNeill KM, and Amy BW. Terrorism coordination: a state-level perspective. In: Johnson JJ, Ledlow GR, and Jones WJ, eds. *Community Preparedness and Response to Terrorism.* vol. I: *The Terrorist Threat to Our Communities.* Westport, CT: Greenwood; 2005.

5. World Health Organization. Reports on global HIV/AIDS situation. Available at: http://www.who.int/hiv/epiupdates/en/index.html. Accessed: Jan. 18, 2010.

6. Mostashari F, Bunning ML, Kitsutani PT, Singer DA, Nash D, Cooper MJ, Katz N, Liljebjelke KA, Biggerstaff BJ, Fine AD, Layton MC, Mullin SM, Johnson AJ, Martin DA, Hayes EB, and Campbell GL. Epidemic West Nile encephalitis, New York, 1999: Results of a household-based seroepidemiological survey. *Lancet.* 2001; 358(9278):261–264.

7. Centers for Disease Control and Prevention. Health care-associated methicillin resistant *Staphylococcus aureus* (HA-MRSA). Available at: http://www.cdc.gov/ ncidod/dhqp/ar_MRSA.html. Accessed: Jan. 18, 2010.

8. WebMD. Understanding MRSA (methicillin resistant *Staphylococcus aureus*). Available at: http://www.webmd.com/skin-problems-and-treatments/understanding-mrsa -methicillin-resistant-staphylococcus-aureus. Accessed: Jan. 18, 2010.

9. Centers for Disease Control and Prevention. BSE (bovine spongiform encephalopathy). Available at: http://www.cdc.gov/ncidod/dvrd/bse. Accessed: Jan. 18, 2010.

10. World Health Organization. Bovine spongiform encephalopathy. Available at: http://www.who.int/mediacentre/factsheets/fs113/en. Accessed: Jan. 18, 2010.

11. Centers for Disease Control and Prevention. Cholera. Available at: http://www.cdc .gov/nczved/dfbmd/disease_listing/cholera_gi.html. Accessed: Jan. 18, 2010.

12. World Health Organization. Cholera. Available at: http://www.who.int/topics/ cholera/en. Accessed: Jan. 21, 2010.

13. Centers for Disease Control and Prevention. Ebola hemorrhagic fever. Available at: http://www.cdc.gov/ncidod/dvrd/spb/mnpages/dispages/Ebola.htm. Accessed: Jan. 21, 2010.

14. World Health Organization. Ebola hemorrhagic fever. Available at: http://www .who.int/mediacentre/factsheets/fs103/en. Accessed: Jan. 21, 2010.

15. Centers for Disease Control and Prevention. E. coli. Available at: http://www.cdc .gov/ecoli. Accessed: Jan. 21, 2010.

16. Centers for Disease Control and Prevention. Preventing group B Strep. Available at: http://www.cdc.gov/GroupBstrep. Accessed: Jan. 22, 2010.

17. Centers for Disease Control and Prevention. Legionellosis resource site. Available at: http://www.cdc.gov/legionella/index.htm. Accessed: Jan. 22, 2010.

18. U.S. National Library of Medicine, Medline Plus. Legionnaires' disease. Available at: http://www.nlm.nih.gov/medlineplus/legionnairesdisease.html. Accessed: Jan. 22, 2010.

19. Centers for Disease Control and Prevention. National Center for Immunization and Respiratory Diseases. Vaccines and preventable diseases: Polio vaccination. Available at: http://www.cdc.gov/vaccines/vpd-vac/polio/default.htm. Accessed: Jan. 24, 2010.

20. Centers for Disease Control and Prevention, Division of Foodborne, Bacterial, and Mycotic Diseases. Salmonellosis. Available at: http://www.cdc.gov/nczved/dfbmd/disease_listing/salmonellosis_gi.html. Accessed: Jan. 24, 2010.

21. Centers for Disease Control and Prevention. Severe acute respiratory syndrome (SARS). Available at: http://www.cdc.gov/ncidod/sars. Accessed: Jan. 24, 2010.

22. U.S. National Library of Medicine, Medline Plus. Tuberculosis. Available at: http://www.nlm.nih.gov/medlineplus/tuberculosis.html. Accessed: Jan. 25, 2010.

23. Centers for Disease Control and Prevention. Emergency preparedness and response: tularemia. Available at: http://www.bt.cdc.gov/agent/tularemia. Accessed: Jan. 25, 2010.

24. Centers for Disease Control and Prevention. H1N1 flu. Available at: http://www.cdc.gov/H1N1flu/qa.htm. Accessed: Jan. 25, 2010.

25. Centers for Disease Control and Prevention. Deaths: Leading causes for 2002. *National Vital Statistics Reports*. 2005; 53(17).

26. Kochanek KD, Murphy SL, Anderson RN, and Scott C. Deaths: Final data for 2002. *National Vital Statistics Reports*. 2004; 53(5).

27. Mackay J and Mensah GA. *The Atlas of Heart Disease and Stroke*. Geneva: World Health Organization; 2004.

28. Zheng ZJ, Croft JB, Giles WH, Ayala C, Greenlund K, Keenan NL, Neff L, Wattigney WA, and Mensah GA. State specific mortality from sudden cardiac death: United States, 1999. *Morbidity and Mortality Weekly Report*. 2002; 51:123–126.

29. *2006 National Hospital Discharge Survey*. Atlanta: Centers for Disease Control and Prevention; 2006.

30. *Death: Final Data for 2005*. Atlanta: Centers for Disease Control and Prevention; 2006.

31. Hootman JM and Helmick CG. Projections of US prevalence of arthritis and associated activity limitations. *Arthritis and Rheumatism*. 2006; 54(1):226–229.

32. Sacks JJ, Helmick CG, and Langmaid G. Deaths from arthritis and other rheumatic conditions, United States, 1979–1998. *Journal of Rheumatology*. 2004; 31:1823–1828.

33. U.S. Cancer Statistics Working Group. *United States Cancer Statistics: 2004 Incidence and Mortality*. Atlanta: U.S. Department of Health and Human Services, Centers for Disease Control and Prevention, and National Cancer Institute; 2007.

34. Ogden CL, Carroll MD, McDowell MA, and Flegal KM. *Obesity Among Adults in the United States—No Change Since 2003–2004*. NCHS data brief No. 1. Hyattsville, MD: National Center for Health Statistics; 2007.

35. Ogden CL, Carroll MD, and Flegal KM. High body mass index for age among US children and adolescents, 2003–2006. *Journal of the American Medical Association*. 2008; 299(20):2401–2405.

36. U.S. Department of Health and Human Services. *Healthy People 2010*. 2nd ed. Washington, DC: Government Printing Office; 2000.

37. Seeff LC, Richards TB, Shapiro JA, Nadel MR, Manninen DL, and Given LS. How many endoscopies are performed for colorectal cancer screening? Results of the CDC's survey of endoscopic capacity. *Gastroenterology*. 2004; 127:1670–1677.

38. U.S. National Institutes of Health, National Cancer Institute. SEER stat fact sheets: cervix uteri. Available at: http://seer.cancer.gov/statfacts/html/cervix.html. Accessed: Jan. 25, 2010.

39. Ries LAG, Melbert D, Krapcho M, Mariotto A, Miller BA, Feuer EJ, Clegg L, Horner MJ, Howlader N, Eisner MP, Reichman M, and Edwards BK, eds. *SEER Cancer Statistics Review, 1975–2004*. Bethesda, MD: National Cancer Institute: 2007.

40. U.S. National Institutes of Health, National Cancer Institute. The prostate cancer outcomes study: fact sheet. Available at: http://www.cancer.gov/cancertopics/ factsheet/support/pcos. Accessed: Jan. 25, 2010.

41. Bostwick DG, Burke HB, Djakiew D, Euling S, Ho S, Landolph J, Bostwick DG, Burke HB, Djakiew D, Euling S, Ho SM, Landolph J, Morrison H, Sonawane B, Shifflett T, Waters DJ, and Timms B. Human prostate cancer risk factors. *Cancer* 2004; 101(10 Suppl):2371–2490.

42. U.S. National Institutes of Health, National Cancer Institute. Skin cancer. Available at: http://www.cancer.gov/cancertopics/types/skin. Accessed: Jan. 25, 2010.

43. National Institutes of Health. *What You Need to Know About Skin Cancer*. Government Printing Office; 2005. NIH publication No. 05–1564.

44. Centers for Disease Control and Prevention. Asthma Data Surveillance. Available at: http://www.cdc.gov/asthma/asthmadata.htm. Accessed: Jan. 12, 2010.

45. National Heart, Lung, and Blood Institute. Asthma Data and Surveillance. Available at: http://www.nhlbi.nih.gov/health/prof/lung/asthma/surveil.htm. Accessed: Jan. 15, 2010.

46. Centers for Disease Control and Prevention. Behavioral Risk Factor Surveillance Survey. Available at: http://www.cdc.gov/ASTHMA/brfss/default.htm. Accessed: Jan. 12, 2010.

Note: *Pages numbers in italic are for figures or tables*